Equine Neonatology

Editor

PAMELA A. WILKINS

VETERINARY CLINICS OF NORTH AMERICA: EQUINE PRACTICE

www.vetequine.theclinics.com

Consulting Editor
THOMAS J. DIVERS

December 2015 • Volume 31 • Number 3

ELSEVIER

1600 John F. Kennedy Boulevard • Suite 1800 • Philadelphia, Pennsylvania, 19103-2899

http://www.vetequine.theclinics.com

VETERINARY CLINICS OF NORTH AMERICA: EQUINE PRACTICE Volume 31, Number 3
December 2015 ISSN 0749-0739, ISBN-13: 978-0-323-40276-7

Editor: Patrick Manley
Developmental Editor: Donald Mumford

Veterinary Clinics of North America: Equine Practice (ISSN 0749-0739) is published in April, August, and December by Elsevier Inc., 360 Park Avenue South, New York, NY 10010-1710. Business and Editorial Offices: 1600 John F. Kennedy Blvd., Suite 1800, Philadelphia, PA 19103-2899. Subscription prices are $270.00 per year (domestic individuals), $431.00 per year (domestic institutions), $130.00 per year (domestic students/residents), $315.00 per year (Canadian individuals), $543.00 per year (Canadian institutions), $365.00 per year (international individuals), $543.00 per year (international institutions), and $180.00 per year (international and Canadian students/residents). To receive student/resident rate, orders must be accompanied by name of affiliated institution, date of term, and the signature of program/residency coordinator on institution letterhead. Orders will be billed at individual rate until proof of status is received. Foreign air speed delivery is included in all *Clinics* subscription prices. All prices are subject to change without notice. **POSTMASTER:** Send address changes to *Veterinary Clinics of North America: Equine Practice*, 3251 Riverport Lane, Maryland Heights, MO 63043. Customer Service (orders, claims, online, change of address): Elsevier Health Sciences Division, Subscription **Customer Service, 3251 Riverport Lane, Maryland Heights, MO 63043. Tel: 1-800-654-2452 (U.S. and Canada); 314-447-8871 (outside U.S. and Canada). Fax: 314-447-8029. E-mail: journalscustomerservice-usa@elsevier.com (for print support);** E-mail: **journalsonlinesupport-usa@elsevier. com (for online support)**.

Reprints. For copies of 100 or more of articles in this publication, please contact the Commercial Reprints Department, Elsevier Inc., 360 Park Avenue South, New York, NY 10010-1710. Tel.: 212-633-3874; Fax: 212-633-3820; E-mail: reprints@elsevier.com.

Veterinary Clinics of North America: Equine Practice is covered in *MEDLINE/PubMed (Index Medicus)*, *Excerpta Medica*, *Current Contents/Agriculture, Biology and Environmental Sciences*, and *ISI*.

Printed in the United States of America.

Contributors

CONSULTING EDITOR

THOMAS J. DIVERS, DVM
Diplomate, American College of Veterinary Internal Medicine; Diplomate, American College of Veterinary Emergency and Critical Care; Steffen Professor of Veterinary Medicine, Section Chief, Section of Large Animal Medicine, College of Veterinary Medicine, Cornell University, Ithaca, New York

EDITOR

PAMELA A. WILKINS, BS, DVM, MS, PhD
Diplomate, American College of Veterinary Internal Medicine-Large Animal; Diplomate, American College of Veterinary Emergency and Critical Care; Professor of Equine Internal Medicine, Department of Veterinary Clinical Medicine, University of Illinois College of Veterinary Medicine, Urbana-Champaign, Urbana, Illinois

AUTHORS

STUART CLARK-PRICE, DVM, MS
Diplomate, American College of Veterinary Internal Medicine; Diplomate, American College of Veterinary Anesthesia and Analgesia; Assistant Professor of Anesthesia and Pain Management, Clinical Service Head, Anesthesia and Pain Management; Department of Veterinary Clinical Medicine, College of Veterinary Medicine, University of Illinois, Urbana, Illinois

CHRISTOPHER LANGDON FIELDING, DVM
Diplomate, American College of Veterinary and Critical Care; Diplomate, American College of Veterinary Sports Medicine and Rehabilitation; Loomis Basin Equine Medical Center, Penryn, California

BERIT FISCHER, DVM
Diplomate, Amercian College of Veterinary Anesthesia and Analgesia; Service Head, Department of Anesthesia and Pain Management, Animal Medical Center New York, New York

STEPHEN JOSLYN, BSc, BVMS, MRCVS
Diplomate, European College of Veterinary Diagnostic Imaging; Clinical Assistant Professor, Department of Veterinary Clinical Medicine, University of Illinois College of Veterinary Medicine, Urbana, Illinois

KARA M. LASCOLA, DVM, MS
Diplomate, American College of Veterinary Medicine – Large Animal Internal Medicine; Assistant Professor, Department of Veterinary Clinical Medicine, University of Illinois College of Veterinary Medicine, Urbana, Illinois

DAVID G. LEVINE, DVM
Diplomate, American College of Veterinary Surgeons; Assistant Professor of Clinical Large Animal Surgery, University of Pennsylvania, Philadelphia, Pennsylvania

KIRAGOS GARY MAGDESIAN, DVM
Diplomate, American College of Veterinary Internal Medicine; Diplomate, American College of Veterinary and Critical Care; Diplomate, American College of Veterinary Clinical Pharmacology; Henry Endowed Chair in Critical Care and Emergency Medicine, School of Veterinary Medicine, University of California, Davis, Davis, California

CELIA M. MARR, BVMS, MVM, PhD
RCVS Diplomate, Equine Internal Medicine; Diplomate, European College of Equine Internal Medicine; Rossdales Equine Hospital and Diagnostic Centre, Suffolk, United Kingdom

ASHLEIGH V. MORRICE, BSc, DVM
Equine Centre, Faculty of Veterinary and Agricultural Sciences, The University of Melbourne, Werribee, Victoria, Australia

STEPHEN REED, DVM
Diplomate, American College of Veterinary Internal Medicine; Rood and Riddle Equine Hospital, Lexington, Kentucky

KIM A. SPRAYBERRY, DVM
Diplomate, American College of Veterinary Internal Medicine; Animal Science Department, Cal Poly University San Luis Obispo, San Luis Obispo, California

BRETT S. TENNENT-BROWN, BSc, DipSc, BVSc, MS
Diplomate, American College of Veterinary Internal Medicine; Diplomate, American College of Veterinary Emergency and Critical Care; Equine Centre, Faculty of Veterinary and Agricultural Sciences, The University of Melbourne, Werribee, Victoria, Australia

PAMELA A. WILKINS, BS, DVM, MS, PhD
Diplomate, American College of Veterinary Internal Medicine-Large Animal; Diplomate, American College of Veterinary Emergency and Critical Care; Professor of Equine Internal Medicine, Department of Veterinary Clinical Medicine, University of Illinois College of Veterinary Medicine, Urbana-Champaign, Urbana, Illinois

DAVID M. WONG, DVM, MS
Diplomate, American College of Veterinary Internal Medicine; Diplomate, American College of Veterinary Emergency and Critical Care; Department of Veterinary Clinical Sciences, Lloyd Veterinary Medical Center, College of Veterinary Medicine, Iowa State University, Ames, Iowa

Contents

Defining and describing the systemic inflammatory response syndrome (SIRS) and sepsis has facilitated recognition and investigation of the complex disease processes involving the host response to infection and trauma. Over the years a variety of definitions of SIRS have been examined and applied to numerous research studies to improve critical care in both human and veterinary clinical practice. This article summarizes the history of the development of the SIRS definition, outlines the pathophysiologic processes that are involved in SIRS, and provides a specific definition for use in foal medicine.

Sepsis and septic shock represent a major cause of morbidity and mortality in equine neonates and in all species. Early recognition of the condition is important, but definitive examination and laboratory variables to predict equine neonatal sepsis are lacking. Early and aggressive treatment should include broad-spectrum antimicrobial coverage, source control, and hemodynamic support. Field practitioners and intensive care clinicians work together in the management of this condition because the recognition and initial treatment should begin as early as possible.

Diagnostic imaging plays an essential role in the diagnosis and monitoring of lower respiratory disease in neonatal foals. Radiography is most widely available to equine practitioners and is the primary modality that has been used for the characterization of respiratory disease in foals. Computed tomography imaging, although still limited in availability to the general practitioner, offers advantages over radiography and has been used diagnostically in neonatal foals with respiratory disease. Recognition of appropriate imaging protocols and patient-associated artifacts is critical for accurate image interpretation regardless of the modality used.

Diagnostic imaging can substantially augment physical examination findings in neonatal foals. Used in combination with radiography or as a stand-alone imaging modality, ultrasound evaluation of the thoracic and abdominal body cavities can be a high-yield diagnostic undertaking. Many of the conditions that afflict neonatal foals are highly amenable to sonographic interrogation, including pneumonia and other changes in the lungs associated with sepsis, systemic inflammatory response syndrome, multiple organ dysfunction, and prematurity; colic arising from medical and surgical causes; and urinary tract disorders. Sonographic imaging is not impaired by intracavitary fluid accumulation and reveals abnormalities of soft tissue and bony origin.

 Videos pertaining to the equine neonatal cardiovascular system accompany this article

The neonatal foal is in a transitional state from prenatal to postnatal circulation. Healthy newborn foals often have cardiac murmurs and dysrhythmias, which are usually transient and of little clinical significance. The neonatal foal is prone to infection and cardiac trauma. Echocardiography is the main tool used for valuation of the cardiovascular system. With prompt identification and appropriate action, dysrhythmias and other sequel to cardiac trauma can be corrected. With infection, the management and prognosis are driven by concurrent sepsis. Congenital disease represents an interesting diagnostic challenge for the neonatologist, but surgical correction is not appropriate for most equids.

Anesthetizing the neonatal foal presents significant challenges as a result of physiologic differences from the adult equine. This article gives the reader an overview of these differences and the impact they have on anesthetic drug selection, monitoring, and support of the equine neonate. Special emphasis is directed to the sick neonate and appropriate preparation and maintenance of anesthesia in the face of commonly presented disease conditions.

Neonatal encephalopathy is the most common neurologic condition affecting newborn foals and shares similarities with perinatal asphyxia syndrome of human infants. However, in many cases of neonatal encephalopathy there is no obvious episode of acute or chronic hypoxia and other mechanisms likely play a role in the pathogenesis. Increased concentrations of neuroactive progestagens are found in affected foals; whether these molecules are protective, as has been suggested, or play a role in the pathogenesis is unknown. Neurologic diseases other than neonatal encephalopathy affect foals occasionally and should be considered when evaluating sick foals with clinical signs of neurologic dysfunction.

The first weeks of life are critical in many aspects, and the musculoskeletal system is no exception. Being able to stand and nurse within hours of life is necessary for survival. Laxity, flexural deformities, and skeletal immaturity can all make it difficult for neonates to ambulate. The increased vascularity to bones and cartilage mixed with the newly forming immune system also make neonates susceptible to infections that we rarely see in adult animals. This article concentrates on orthopedic conditions seen in the first 2 weeks of life.

Equine neonatal intensive care units have expanded knowledge and understanding of the normal and abnormal physiology of the equine neonate, resulting in successful treatment of critically ill equine neonates. The overall survival rate has increased tremendously since the early 1980s, from a little more than 50% to 80% or more for most facilities. The severely septic foal and the very premature foal still remain large treatment challenges, but less severely septic foals and foals challenged by adverse peripartum events such as dystocia and placentitis are surviving to hospital discharge and performing to the owners' expectation in larger numbers.

VETERINARY CLINICS OF NORTH AMERICA: EQUINE PRACTICE

THE CLINICS ARE NOW AVAILABLE ONLINE!
Access your subscription at:
www.theclinics.com

Preface

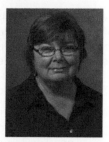

Pamela A. Wilkins, BS, DVM, MS, PhD
Editor

The application of principles and standards of the practice of equine neonatology continues to improve our ability to provide excellent care to sick foals, both in the field and at referral hospitals. The expansion of our knowledge of these small patients is rapid and, as I tell the veterinary students, interns, residents, and equine practitioners I enjoy interacting with, half of what I teach now will be different in 10 years; I just do not yet know which half! It is impossible to present all the most recent advances in equine neonatology in one issue, so what we have done for this issue is focus on a few concepts and technology applications that are advancing our ability to accurately diagnose and manage these patients more efficiently. The authors of articles in this issue are acknowledged as experts in their fields and dedicate their time and energy not just to evolving the science but also to sharing gained knowledge to those of us in equine practice at every opportunity.

I am grateful to Dr Tom Divers, a living legend, for the opportunity to guest edit this issue, and to Patrick Manley and Donald Mumford from Elsevier for their support in the process. I would particularly like to acknowledge those who contributed so meaningfully to my sometimes circuitous career pathway by providing support, training me to think critically both in and outside the box, and demonstrating what true critique and collegiality look like. This list is too long to publish here, but you all know who you are. I am still trying to pay it forward and to "lean in"! We stand on the shoulders of those who came before us.

Finally, I need to thank the owners, referring veterinarians, practitioners, breeders, trainers, and research foundations who have supported all the work done by so many to advance our ability to treat the foals we all care about so much. Without you, we would not be where we are now. We are ever grateful.

Pamela A. Wilkins, BS, DVM, MS, PhD
Professor of Equine Internal Medicine
College of Veterinary Medicine
Department of Veterinary Clinical Medicine
University of Illinois
1008 West Hazelwood Drive
Urbana, IL 61801, USA

E-mail address:
pawilkin@illinois.edu

Defining the Systemic Inflammatory Response Syndrome in Equine Neonates

 CrossMark

David M. Wong, DVM, MS[a],*, Pamela A. Wilkins, BS, DVM, MS, PhD[b]

KEYWORDS

- SIRS • Sepsis • Organ dysfunction • Foal • Endotoxemia

KEY POINTS

- The systemic inflammatory response syndrome (SIRS) definition originated because of a need to improve recognition, diagnosis, monitoring, and treatment of sepsis and its sequelae (multiple organ dysfunction).
- SIRS is most commonly initiated by infection, but other disease processes, such as trauma, burns, sterile inflammatory conditions, severe hemorrhage, or surgery can also result in SIRS.
- The pathophysiology of SIRS is primarily mediated by cytokines and involves complex interactions involving the host's immune, hemostatic, cardiovascular, nervous, and endocrine systems.
- SIRS has been variably defined and applied in a limited number of equine studies. Defining specific SIRS criteria is vital to future investigations of disease processes, particularly sepsis, of both foals and adult horses in order to allow reasonable and accurate comparison of studies designed to improve veterinary care of these vulnerable patients.

The original intent for establishing the definition of the systemic inflammatory response syndrome (SIRS) along with sepsis, severe sepsis, and septic shock was to provide clinicians with a clinically relevant guide for identification, treatment, and monitoring of septic patients and to allow standardization of inclusion criteria for patients participating in research protocols and clinical trials. Essentially, definitions were developed to facilitate early identification of sepsis and to allow meaningful comparisons so that interventions could be appropriately judged by outcome

Disclosure: The authors have nothing to disclose.
[a] Department of Veterinary Clinical Sciences, Lloyd Veterinary Medical Center, College of Veterinary Medicine, Iowa State University, Ames, IA 50036, USA; [b] Department of Veterinary Clinical Medicine, College of Veterinary Medicine, University of Illinois at Urbana-Champaign, Urbana, IL 61802, USA
* Corresponding author.
E-mail address: DWONG@IASTATE.EDU

criteria. Since the published inception, the concept of SIRS has inundated the medical literature and has been commonly used in medical research and clinical practice, sometimes without regard for important species and age-related differences. However, as the SIRS concept evolved, it became apparent that the definition of both SIRS and sepsis needed refining. Furthermore, a specific definition of SIRS has not been established for equine medicine. This article outlines the history and pathophysiology of SIRS and suggests specific standardized parameters that can be used in foals.

HISTORY OF THE SYSTEMIC INFLAMMATORY RESPONSE SYNDROME

The general concept of articulating SIRS to describe the complex pathophysiologic proinflammatory response to a variety of insults originated from the 1991 Consensus Conference held by the American College of Chest Physicians and Society of Critical Care Medicine.[1] Infection was thought to be the primary initiator of SIRS, but alternative insults such as trauma, burns, sterile inflammatory processes (eg, pancreatitis), hemorrhagic shock, severe surgery, or other proinflammatory conditions were also thought to result in SIRS.[1,2] The conference participants were charged with the task of establishing definitions that could be applied to patients with sepsis and its sequelae (eg, sepsis-associated organ dysfunction) and that would serve to improve the ability of clinicians to diagnose, monitor, and treat sepsis.[1] More specifically, the intent was to provide a conceptual and clinically practical framework to define progressive injury generally termed sepsis and sepsis-associated organ dysfunction.[1,3] A further goal was to create an easily applied set of clinical parameters that would allow for early bedside detection of sepsis, thereby allowing early therapeutic intervention.[1] These definitions and clinical parameters were also intended to facilitate dissemination of applicable information garnered from clinical studies with more standardized research protocols, and allow early detection of potential candidates for clinical trials investigating therapeutic strategies for sepsis.[1,4] As a result of that conference, broad definitions of sepsis, SIRS, and the physiologic parameters used to categorize patients was published. These definitions were widely incorporated into clinical practice, clinical trials, and medical research, and they remain clinically relevant (Box 1).

The definition of SIRS satisfied a clinical need for a diagnostic tool that could be applied by most hospitals, regardless of size or location. In light of this, the definition of SIRS did not require specific sophisticated or time-consuming diagnostic tests, but maintained a reasonable degree of certainty in identifying patients with possible sepsis.[4] The SIRS parameters are sensitive, developed to include all potential patients with a proinflammatory response. However, the criteria lack specificity for a particular clinical disorder or the presence of infection and were viewed skeptically by some clinicians and researchers.[5,6] In 2001, another consensus conference sponsored by several international intensive care societies revisited the 1991 consensus definitions with 3 specific goals: (1) to review strengths and weakness of the current definitions of sepsis and related conditions; (2) to identify ways to improve those definitions; and (3) to identify methodologies that improved the accuracy, reliability, and/or clinical utility for the diagnosis of sepsis.[3] The members of the 2001 Consensus Conference stated that the SIRS concept is valid in the sense that systemic inflammation can be triggered by a variety of infectious and noninfectious conditions, but the definition of SIRS was overly sensitive and nonspecific to be useful in diagnosing a cause of the syndrome or identifying a distinct pattern of host response.[3,6,7] Subsequently, conference members suggested that biochemical parameters and inflammatory mediators, such as

---

Box 1
Definitions from the American College of Chest Physicians and Society of Critical Care Medicine Consensus Conference

- Bacteremia: the presence of viable bacteria in the blood.

- Infection: microbial phenomenon characterized by an inflammatory response to the presence of microorganisms or the invasion of normally sterile host tissue by those organisms.

- SIRS in adults: the systemic inflammatory response to a variety of severe clinical insults. The response is manifested by 2 or more of the following conditions:
  - Temperature greater than 38°C (100.4°F) or less than 36°C (96.8°F)
  - Heart rate greater than 90 beats per minute
  - Respiratory rate greater than 20 breaths per minute or $Paco_2$ less than 32 mm Hg
  - White blood cell count greater than 12,000/mm³, less than 4000/mm³, or more than 10% immature (band) forms

- Sepsis: the systemic response to infection, manifested by 2 or more of the aforementioned SIRS criteria listed immediately above.

- Severe sepsis: sepsis associated with organ dysfunction, hypoperfusion, or hypotension.[a] Hypoperfusion and perfusion abnormalities may include, but are not limited to, lactic acidosis, oliguria, or an acute alteration in mental status.

- Septic shock: sepsis-induced hypotension despite adequate fluid resuscitation along with the presence of perfusion abnormalities that may include, but are not limited to, lactic acidosis, oliguria, or an acute alteration in mental status. Patients who are receiving inotropic or vasopressor agents may not be hypotensive at the time that perfusion abnormalities are measured.

- Sepsis-induced hypotension: a systolic blood pressure less than 90 mm Hg or a reduction of greater than or equal to 40 mm Hg from baseline in the absence of other causes of hypotension.

- Multiple organ dysfunction syndrome (MODS): presence of altered organ function in an acutely ill patient such that homeostasis cannot be maintained without intervention.

[a] Hypotension defined by Systolic arterial pressure less than 90 mm Hg; mean arterial pressure less than 60 mm Hg, or reduction of systolic blood pressure of more than 40 mm Hg from baseline, despite adequate volume resuscitation, in the absence of other causes of hypotension.[1,3]

Adapted from Bone RC, Balk RA, Cerra FB, et al. Definitions for sepsis and organ failure and guidelines for the use of innovative therapies in sepsis. The AACP/SCCM Consensus Conference Committee. American College of Chest Physicians/Society of Critical Care Medicine. Chest 1992;101:1646; and Goldstein B, Giroir B, Randolph A, et al. International Pediatric Sepsis Consensus Conference: definitions for sepsis and organ dysfunction in pediatrics. Pediatr Crit Care Med 2005;6:2–8; with permission.

---

interleukin (IL)-6, adrenomedullin, soluble cluster of differentiation 14 (CD14), and C-reactive protein may be more consistent and should be used to identify the inflammatory response, but large prospective studies investigating the association between SIRS and these biomarkers were needed. Although the definitions of infection, sepsis, severe sepsis, and septic shock remained largely unchanged, one change from the 1991 consensus statement was a list of possible signs of systemic inflammation, specifically in response to infection, that provide physical and laboratory abnormalities that would prompt an experienced clinician to conclude that the infected patient looks septic.[3] The primary issue debated was the importance of an accurate bedside diagnosis of sepsis versus entry criteria for clinical trials because participants thought that facilitating bedside diagnosis should have priority.

The 1991 and 2001 Consensus Conferences based the SIRS criteria on clinical signs and laboratory values in adults and was intended for use in the adult population.[1,3] In contrast, little guidance or consensus was available for the definition of pediatric SIRS with infection (pediatric sepsis). In 2002, international experts in adult and pediatric sepsis (International Pediatric Sepsis Consensus Conference) gathered with the goal of evaluating and establishing SIRS criteria in pediatric patients along with creating consensus definitions of pediatric infection, sepsis, severe sepsis, septic shock, and multiple organ dysfunction syndrome (MODS).[8] The Consensus Committee recognized that physiologic parameters change as children age and that clinical variables used to define SIRS and organ dysfunction need to be adjusted accordingly, based on age-specific vital parameters and laboratory data documented in healthy children.[8] Centered on this premise, 6 specific pediatric age groups were recommended: newborn (0 days to 1 week), neonate (1 week to 1 month), infant (1 month to 1 year), toddler and preschool (2–5 years), school age (6–12 years), and adolescent and young adult (13 to <18 years).[8] The specific definitions put forth by the Consensus Committee are listed in **Boxes 2** and **3**.

A notable difference between pediatric and adult definitions is that pediatric SIRS required that either temperature or leukocyte abnormalities be present to fulfill the

---

Box 2
Definitions of SIRS, infection, sepsis, severe sepsis, and septic shock from the International Pediatric Sepsis Consensus Conference

- Infection: a suspected or proven (by positive blood culture, tissue stain, or polymerase chain reaction test) infection caused by any pathogen, or a clinical syndrome associated with a high probability of infection. Evidence of infection includes positive findings on clinical examination, imaging, or laboratory tests (eg, white blood cells in a normally sterile body fluid, perforated viscus, chest radiograph consistent with pneumonia, petechial or purpuric rash, or purpura fulminans).

- SIRS in children: the presence of at least 2 of the following 4 criteria, 1 of which must be abnormal temperature or leukocyte count:
  o Core temperature of greater than 38.5°C (101.3°F) or less than 36°C (96.8°F)
  o Tachycardia, as defined as a mean heart rate of more than 2 standard deviations (SD) greater than the normal for age in the absence of external stimulus, chronic drugs, or painful stimuli; or otherwise unexplained persistent increase for a 0.5-hour to 4-hour time period; or, for children less than 1 year old, bradycardia, defined as a mean heart rate less than the tenth percentile for age in the absence of external vagal stimulus, β-blocker drugs, or congenital heart disease; or otherwise unexplained persistent depression for 0.5-hour time period
  o Mean respiratory rate more than 2 SD greater than normal for age, or mechanical ventilation for an acute process not related to an underlying neuromuscular disease, or administration of general anesthesia
  o Leukocyte count increased or depressed for age (not secondary to chemotherapy-induced leucopenia) or more than 10% immature neutrophils

- Sepsis: SIRS in the presence of, or as a result of, suspected or proven infection.

- Severe sepsis: sepsis plus one of the following: cardiovascular organ dysfunction, or acute respiratory distress syndrome, or 2 or more other organ dysfunctions (respiratory, renal, neurologic, hematologic, or hepatic). Organ dysfunctions are defined in **Box 3**.

- Septic shock: sepsis and cardiovascular organ dysfunction as defined in **Box 3**.

From Goldstein B, Giroir B, Randolph A, et al. International Pediatric Sepsis Consensus Conference: definitions for sepsis and organ dysfunction in pediatrics. Pediatr Crit Care Med 2005;6:4; with permission.

Box 3
Organ dysfunction criteria (pediatric) from the International Pediatric Sepsis Consensus Conference

Cardiovascular dysfunction: despite administration of isotonic intravenous fluid bolus greater than or equal to 40 mL/kg in 1 hour:

- Decrease blood pressure (hypotension) to less than the fifth percentile for age or systolic blood pressure less than 2 SD less than normal for age, or

- Need for vasoactive drug to maintain blood pressure in normal range (dopamine >5 µg/kg/min; or dobutamine, epinephrine, or norepinephrine at any dose), or

- Two of the following:
  - Unexplained metabolic acidosis: base deficit greater than 5.0 mEq/L
  - Increased arterial lactate level greater than 2 times upper limit of normal
  - Oliguria: urine output less than 0.5 mL/kg/h
  - Prolonged capillary refill: greater than 5 seconds
  - Core to peripheral temperature gap greater than $3°C$

Respiratory dysfunction

- Pao_2/fraction of inspired oxygen (Fio_2) less than 300 in absence of cyanotic heart disease or preexisting lung disease, or

- $Paco_2$ more than 20 mm Hg (65 torr) greater than baseline $Paco_2$, or

- Proven need or greater than 50% Fio_2 to maintain saturation greater than or equal to 92%, or

- Need for nonelective invasive or noninvasive mechanical ventilation

Neurologic dysfunction

- Glasgow Come Score less than or equal to 11, or

- Acute change in mental status with a decrease in Glasgow Coma Score greater than or equal to 3 points from abnormal baseline

Hematologic dysfunction

- Platelet count less than 80,000/mm^3 or a decline of 50% in platelet count from highest value recorded over the past 3 days (for chronic hematology/oncology patients), or

- International Normalized Ratio greater than 2

Renal dysfunction

- Serum creatinine greater than or equal to 2 times upper limit of normal for age or 2-fold increase in baseline creatinine level

Hepatic dysfunction

- Total bilirubin 4 mg/dL (not applicable for newborn), or

- Alanine aminotransferase level 2 times upper limit of normal for age

From Goldstein B, Giroir B, Randolph A, et al. International Pediatric Sepsis Consensus Conference: definitions for sepsis and organ dysfunction in pediatrics. Pediatr Crit Care Med 2005;6:5; with permission.

pediatric SIRS criteria.[1,3,8] The basis of this recommendation was that several disease processes in the pediatric population present with tachycardia and tachypnea.[8] Other differences between the pediatric and adult definitions included the stipulation that numeric values for each criterion be modified to account for different physiology of children as they age and that bradycardia be recognized as a possible sign of SIRS in newborns, but not in older children.[1,3,8] In addition, fever could be documented by a reliable source at home if measured within 4 hours of presentation to the hospital. Examples of clinical abnormalities indicating infection were described and included petechia and purpura in the setting of hemodynamic instability; fever, cough, and hypoxemia in the setting of leukocytosis and pulmonary infiltrates; and a distended, tympanitic abdomen with fever and leukocytosis associated with a perforated bowel.[8] In children, the definition of septic shock is confounded by children often maintaining blood pressure until they are severely ill[8,9]; shock may therefore occur long before hypotension occurs in children. As a result, there was no requirement for systemic hypotension for the diagnosis of septic shock in children.[8] The consensus statement members also defined pediatric organ dysfunction, aiming to identify reproducible assessments of organ dysfunction that allowed temporal tracking (improvement or deterioration) as potential end points in clinical trials. The members thought that there was a lack of evidence of validity to use the adult organ dysfunction criteria in children. Therefore, the panel developed criteria for organ dysfunction based on several scoring systems.[8,10–13]

PATHOPHYSIOLOGY OF SYSTEMIC INFLAMMATORY RESPONSE SYNDROME

The provision of both adult and pediatric definitions of SIRS, sepsis, severe sepsis, and septic shock allowed clinicians to more easily categorize ill patients in a semiobjective manner and provided guidelines and criteria for research protocols and clinical trials. However, the physiology of inflammation and the pathogenesis of SIRS are highly complex, and in many aspects not fully understood.[14] The body's response to infection or injury involves tightly controlled interactions between proinflammatory and antiinflammatory mediators and the immune, hemostatic, cardiovascular, nervous, and endocrine systems. These interactions participate in a fine balance in which the host's protective response to infection or injury and activation of the immune system can be simultaneously mirrored by hyperactivation of proinflammatory responses and immunosuppression that can be detrimental to the host.[15,16] In general, proinflammatory reactions of the host intended to eliminate infection are thought to be responsible for collateral tissue damage, whereas antiinflammatory responses, needed for limiting local and systemic tissue injury, have been implicated in enhanced host susceptibility to secondary infections.[17]

In an elegant commentary, Fry[17] conceptually summarized the physiologic purpose of the local inflammatory response as a natural mechanism to eradicate infection and contain tissue injury at the local vicinity of the initiating stimulus, while still maintaining the local inflammatory response. In this scheme, the innate immune response is the first line of defense to injury and can be initiated by invasion with microorganisms or tissue injury to the host. Subsequently, disruption of cells and extracellular matrix may occur and result in activation of a variety of endogenous host mechanisms and release or exposure of a variety of mediators. The activity of these mediators promotes the vasoactive and phagocytic phases of inflammation, but, if left unbridled, can result in SIRS. The vasoactive phase of inflammation establishes a local environment within the infected or traumatized area and assists in mobilization and infiltration of phagocytic cells. Vasodilation occurs from mediators (eg, bradykinin, histamine, inducible nitric oxide synthase, cyclooxygenase-2) that increase blood flow while simultaneously slowing blood flow velocity to the affected area.[17–19] Along with increased expression of adhesion molecules, this facilitates margination of leukocytes to the affected region.[18,20] Increased vascular permeability also facilitates leukocyte margination, and the creation of local edema facilitates an aqueous environment for leukocyte migration through the normally condensed extracellular matrix.[17] The presence of chemokines provides specific signals for leukocyte trafficking into inflamed tissue.[21] In the phagocytic phase of inflammation, upregulation of selectin and adhesion molecules on endothelial cells promotes adherence and margination of circulating neutrophils and monocytes under the influence of chemoattractants.[18,20] Monocytes produce proinflammatory cytokines (eg, tumor necrosis factor alpha [TNF-α], IL-1, IL-6) which affect the robustness of phagocytosis of pathogens and removal of degenerating and dead host cells. This process in which cytokine and chemokine release attracts leukocytes to the local area can also cause local tissue destruction (abscess) or cellular injury (pus), which are necessary by-products of an effective local inflammatory response that can heal host tissues.

The pathophysiology of SIRS and sepsis involves activation of the host's innate immune system.[22] In response to infection or injury, small quantities of cytokines are released into the systemic circulation; this acute response is typically controlled by decreased production of proinflammatory mediators and the release of endogenous antagonists, resulting in homeostasis. If the activation stimulus (bacteria, tissue injury, necrotic cells, ischemia-reperfusion [IR] injury) exceeds the ability of the host to contain the inflammatory response locally, systemic inflammation ensues and can result in injury rather than protection of host tissues. The SIRS can be initiated from a variety of causes, including products released from bacteria, such as occurs with infection, or products from damaged cells released after trauma or IR injury.[23,24] The inflammatory process is activated by immune system recognition of pathogen-associated molecular patterns (PAMPs) associated with invading microorganisms. Examples of PAMPs include lipoteichoic acid (gram-positive bacteria), lipopolysaccharide (gram-negative bacteria), unmethylated C-phosphage-G DNA (gram-negative and gram-positive bacteria), flagellin (bacterial flagellum), peptidoglycan, double-stranded viral RNA, and bacterial DNA.[20–25] Alternatively, host cells can activate the immune system through endogenous products termed damage-associated molecular patterns (DAMPs). Endogenous DAMPs can be passively released from nonphysiologic cell death or actively secreted as alarm signals (alarmins) that warn the host of danger by activating the innate immune system.[22] Alarmins are normal nuclear proteins that are produced from necrotic and physiologically stressed cells.[17,25,26] Key DAMPs include histones, high-mobility group box protein-1, heat shock proteins, glycoproteins, end products of advanced glycation, and extracellular RNA and DNA.[16,22,27]

Cell-associated pattern-recognition receptors (PRRs) recognize PAMPs and DAMPs and activate downstream signaling pathways, resulting in the induction of the innate immune responses and production of inflammatory cytokines, interferon (IFN)-gamma, and other mediators.[28] Mammals have distinct classes of PRRs, including Toll-like receptors (TLRs), C-type lectin receptors, nucleotide-binding domain leucine-rich repeat containing proteins, and retinoic acid–inducible gene-1–like receptors.[16,27,28] On recognition of PAMPs or DAMPs, PRRs initiate signal transduction pathways, including activation of nuclear fact kappa beta (NF-Kβ), mitogen-activated protein kinase, or interferon regulatory factor, which control expression of cytokines, chemokines, and interferons.[16,27] Activation of various intracellular signaling pathways results in the release of numerous proinflammatory cytokines and chemokines, such as TNF-α, IL-1β, IL-2, IL-6, IL-8, IL-12, and IFN.[27,29,30] Although the general beneficial role of these proinflammatory mediators is to initiate defense mechanisms and help protect the host from microbial infection (eg, promote macrophage activation and phagocytosis, enhance cell-mediated immunity, upregulate acute phase protein synthesis), exuberant or unbalanced expression contributes to SIRS.[31–33]

Additional activity during the inflammatory response, intended to eliminate and contain infection, can also be detrimental to the host. For example, the inflammatory response involves activated neutrophils and macrophages that produce reactive oxygen and nitrogen species such as hydrogen peroxide (H_2O_2), hypochlorous acid (HClO), hydroxyl radicals (HO•), nitric oxide (NO•), and peroxynitrite anion (ONOO⁻), which can damage host cells and organs.[14,34] Moreover, cytokines, coupled with increased concentrations of prostaglandins and leukotrienes and transmigration of neutrophils and monocytes, can result in endothelial dysfunction leading to vasodilation and increased capillary permeability.[15] This, in turn, results in leakage of fluid from the vasculature and can be clinically associated with hypotension, hemoconcentration, macromolecular extravasation, and global edema.[15,35,36] Host exposure to PAMPs and DAMPs also results in activation of serine protease systems, including the coagulation and complement cascades.[37] The coagulation system maintains a delicate equilibrium between procoagulant and anticoagulant mechanisms. As a result of the inflammatory process, this equilibrium can be disrupted.[38] For example, IL-1 and TNF-α directly affect endothelial surfaces, resulting in expression of tissue factor on endothelial cells as well as monocytes and macrophages.[39,40] Tissue factor (also referred to as factor III, thromboplastin, or CD142) initiates the extrinsic coagulation pathway by activating factor VII (FVII), and forming tissue factor FVIIa complex, which sequentially results in activation of factor X, factor V, and conversion of prothrombin to thrombin (itself a proinflammatory mediator).[39,40] Proinflammatory cytokines can also disrupt naturally occurring antiinflammatory mediators such as antithrombin and activated protein-C.[39,41] Cumulatively, inflammation can potentially result in the development of coagulopathies contributing to microvascular thrombosis and possibly organ dysfunction (**Fig. 1**).[22,42] The complement system is another rapidly acting serine protease system that serves to identify and target pathogens for lysis and phagocytosis. Excessive activation of complement is a central trigger in the development of sepsis.[43,44] Anaphylatoxin C5a is intensely proinflammatory and interaction with its receptors (C5aR, C5L2) results in inhibition of innate immune signaling pathways and impaired phagocyte function (eg, phagocytosis, chemotaxis, oxidative burst) with its associated neutrophil dysfunction, immunoparalysis, coagulopathy, and multiorgan failure being detrimental to the host.[14,43,44]

The neuroendocrine system is also involved in the inflammatory response. Pain results from inflammatory mediator impact on local somatosensory nerves and reduced threshold for stimulation of nociceptors.[45] The parasympathetic and sympathetic

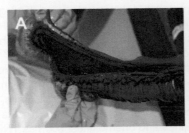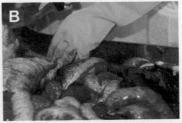

Fig. 1. A 6-day old Percheron filly presented with tachycardia (200 beats/min), tachypnea (60 breaths/min), fever (40.1°C [104.2°F]) and enlarged and patent urachus. Clinical pathology documented leukocytosis (17.66 × 10³/μL), neutrophilia (13.7 × 10³/μL), increased band neutrophils (0.529 × 10³/μL), thrombocytopenia (16 × 10³/μL), and hyperlactatemia (4.9 mmol/L). The foal died 18 hours after presentation. Postmortem examination revealed congestion, hyperemia, and hemorrhage in multiple organs and serosal surfaces (intestinal tract is shown in *A* and *B*) resulting from coagulopathy associated with SIRS/sepsis, likely originating from an infected urachus.

nervous systems also contribute to the immune and inflammatory responses during sepsis and other inflammatory conditions. Afferent reflex arcs sense pathogenic molecules, cytokines, and other products of infection or cell injury and produce action potentials that travel rapidly and specifically to brainstem nuclei.[46] In turn, efferent action potentials travel to immune organs such as the spleen, lymph nodes, and reticuloendothelial organs, and result in release of neurotransmitters that interact with specific receptors on monocytes, macrophages, and lymphocytes.[46] For example, stimulation of the sympathetic nervous system by inflammatory mediators can result in stimulation of adrenergic receptors on macrophages, resulting in enhanced release of cytokines and chemokines, thus intensifying the inflammatory response and SIRS.[14,46–48] In contrast, neural reflexes involving the vagus nerve (so-called neuroinflammatory reflex) causes T cells to release acetylcholine, which interacts with receptors on macrophages to dampen the release of proinflammatory mediators such as TNF-α.[16,47]

Counterbalancing the proinflammatory response is the simultaneous production of antiinflammatory mediators that act to balance the host's need to defend itself against injury while minimizing self-induced tissue damage.[2,49] Antiinflammatory cytokines such as IL-4, IL-5, IL-10, IL-13, and transforming growth factor-β (TGF-β) not only promote the development of humoral immune responses by promoting B-cell differentiation and antibody production but dampen proinflammatory mediators and stimulate immune-regulatory functions.[2,33] For example, IL-10 shows pleiotropic effects, including inhibition of release of TNF-α, IL-1β, and IL-6 from monocytes and macrophages as well as inducing expression of soluble antagonistic proinflammatory receptors IL-1 receptor antagonist (IL-1RA) and soluble TNF receptor, resulting in reduced circulating concentrations of these proinflammatory cytokines.[50–52] A potential consequence of overstimulation of the antiinflammatory pathway is the compensatory antiinflammatory response syndrome (CARS), which can modify the immune status in such a manner that it could favor enhanced susceptibility of the host to infection.[2] Immunosuppressive traits have been observed in septic patients and have been attributed to CARS; characteristic findings in CARS include leukocyte anergy, reduction and apoptosis of lymphocytes, decreased proinflammatory cytokine production, decreased antigen presentation by monocytes, and increased expression of immunosuppressive cytokines.[51,53] Further, increased concentrations of antiinflammatory mediators such as IL-1RA, IL-10, and TNF soluble receptor I and II have been associated with poor outcome and early death in septic models in mice, emphasizing the tight correlation between activation of antiinflammatory signaling and mortality in acute stages of sepsis.[49]

In summary, the inflammatory response can be initiated by a variety of infectious and noninfectious disease processes and involves a multitude of pathways, interactions, and mediators. SIRS is a component of the clinical expression of these varying underlying disease processes. In general, the greater the insult (eg, sepsis, trauma), the greater the response by the host's defense pathways. If the insult is limited, the host responds with a short stress response that is reversed after the damage is corrected. In contrast, if the insult is significant, an overwhelming response is initiated, culminating in SIRS. Uncontrolled progression of SIRS can result in further perturbations in homeostasis and organ function, termed MODS.[1]

THE IMMUNE SYSTEM, SYSTEMIC INFLAMMATORY RESPONSE SYNDROME, AND THE EQUINE NEONATE

Although transient bacteremia can be observed in healthy foals in the early postnatal period ($\leq$12 hours old),[54] sepsis, however defined, remains a leading cause of morbidity and mortality in neonatal foals and is commonly associated with SIRS.[55] The reported incidence of positive bacterial growth in blood cultures collected from ill neonatal foals at admission to referral hospitals ranges from 25.8% to 36% of blood culture samples collected, although the true incidence of sepsis may be higher, as the sensitivity of blood cultures can be low.[55–61] Other diseases associated with SIRS in neonatal foals include perinatal asphyxia syndrome as well as local bacterial infections such as umbilical infections, pneumonia, septic arthritis, or pyelonephritis.[45,60] Before discussing SIRS and sepsis in the foal, a brief comment on the limited knowledge available with regard to cytokine profiles in healthy and ill neonatal foals is indicated.

Mediators associated with SIRS and sepsis have been examined in a limited number of studies involving ill foals.[33,62–64] In one study, expression of TNF-α and TGF-β was significantly lower and expression of IL-8 was significantly greater in blood from sick foals (sick-nonseptic and septic foal groups) compared with healthy foals.[62] In addition, expression of IL-10 was significantly greater in nonsurvivors compared with survivors.[62] In contrast with mouse models, in which increased IL-6, TNF-α, and IL-1β have been measured from septic mice, no significant difference in expression of IL-1β, IL-6, or procalcitonin was noted between sick and healthy foals.[49,62] The investigators suggested that decreased expression of TNF-α in sick foals may relate to TNF-α predominating in early sepsis, but decreases rapidly in the later stages of sepsis.[62,65] The investigators further concluded that the cytokine profile in foals with sepsis may be suggestive of an immunosuppressive state.[62] In a different study by Gold and colleagues,[63] gene expression of IFN-γ, IL-1β, IL-4, IL-6, IL-8, and TLR4 was measured from peripheral blood mononuclear cells (PBMCs) collected from healthy and septic foals at various times during hospitalization. The investigators noted that expression of IL-4 was significantly less in septic foals compared with healthy foals at presentation, but was equivalent between groups by 72 hours.[63] The investigators suggested that healthy neonatal foals might be biased toward an antiinflammatory response (T helper [Th] type 2), but downregulation of gene expression of IL-4 occurs acutely when confronted with an infectious agent.[63] In contrast, another study compared T-cell function in healthy foals by measuring IFN-γ and IL-4 in T-cell subsets, rather than overall cytokine production by PBMCs, to determine Th1 and Th2 responses and documented that healthy foals have an impaired Th2 response and are Th1 biased.[66] Thus, there remains some controversy in the equine literature about Th-cell responses in foals and whether a Th1 or Th2 bias exists.[63,66,67]

Returning to the study by Gold and colleagues,[63] gene expression of TLR4 was significantly increased in septic foals at admission, which may enhance proinflammatory cytokine production. In addition, gene expression of IL-10 was significantly increased in nonsurviving foals, compared with those that survived, similar to the results noted in the study by Pusterla and colleagues.[62,63] Gold and colleagues[63] also noted a 15-fold increase in gene expression of IL-6 in septic foals that died compared with those that survived, but significant differences in IFN-γ, IL-6, or IL-1β were not detected between septic and healthy foals. In a study by Burton and colleagues,[33] septic foals had significantly lower IL-6 concentrations compared with healthy foals; IL-6 concentrations were 47-fold to 62-fold higher in healthy foals compared with septic foals. Note that equine colostrum contains large amounts of IL-6, whereas presuckle serum samples from healthy foals had undetectable IL-6 concentrations before ingestion of colostrum.[33] The investigators suggested that the IL-6 concentration in septic foals was notably lower, compared with healthy foals, because of lack of ingestion of colostrum (ie, failure of passive transfer) in septic foals.[33] Compared with previously noted studies,[62,63] a more recent study documented increased IL-1 gene expression in septic foals; however, IFN-γ gene expression did not differ between healthy and septic foals.[64]

Based on the discordant results in the sparse number of equine neonatal studies, equine clinicians must exercise caution in extrapolating information with regard to sepsis between different age groups and species. Moreover, equine clinicians must recognize that the development of the foal's immune system is complex and not fully understood, and dramatically changes and matures over the first months of life. These changes make interpretation of immune functions and commonly used cytokine and immune cell profiles (ie, inflammatory vs antiinflammatory cytokines, Th1 vs Th2 responses) more difficult when comparing healthy foals with ill foals, foals with adult horses, or foals with other species.[67] As noted earlier, before colostrum ingestion, healthy neonatal foal serum does not contain detectable concentrations of inflammatory cytokines IL-6 or TNF-α[67]; however, measurable amounts of these cytokines are present in colostrum and foal serum after the foal suckles from the mare.[33,68] Note that IL-10, an antiinflammatory cytokine, is not present in colostrum around the time of foaling.[33] Collectively, it has been speculated that the presence of inflammatory mediators (IL-6, TNF-α) and the absence of antiinflammatory mediators (IL-10) within the colostrum promotes cytokine transfer to the foal that is selective and bolsters an inflammatory response, which may increase the overall immune alertness of the newborn foal.[67] However, the true mechanism by which passively transferred maternal cytokines affect the newborn immune system is unknown. In light of this information, interpretation of cytokine profiles in both healthy and ill foals must consider that cytokines are partially passively derived from colostrum and not simply produced by the foal in response to infection and inflammation. Furthermore, cytokines during SIRS and sepsis vary depending on the causative pathogen, phase of disease, and host (eg, genetic) characteristics.[16] There is a clear need for further studies of the inflammatory and antiinflammatory mediators involved in equine neonatal sepsis.

The SIRS concept has been used to categorize both adult horses and foals in equine studies investigating therapeutics, coagulation parameters, or other biomarkers (lactate, glucose) in a variety of disease processes.[60,61,69–74] The first documented use of the SIRS criteria in equine medicine (1999) was applied to a study of hypotensive critically ill foals.[72] Recommended SIRS parameters were based on the 1991 consensus statement in people and centered on perturbations of the total white cell count, body temperature, heart rate, and respiratory rate.[72] The study population consisted of neonatal foals that received norepinephrine infusion to treat hypotension. Subsequently, the SIRS definition was retrospectively applied to identify systemic inflammation (6 of 7 foals) and sepsis (infection plus SIRS). In addition, septic shock (3 of 7 foals) was documented based on positive blood culture, hypotension (mean arterial pressure <60 mm Hg), and the presence of SIRS. The SIRS definition helped categorize neonatal foals with sepsis and septic shock in a retrospective fashion.[72] In other studies, SIRS criteria have been used to investigate associations between systemic inflammation and blood lactate or glucose concentrations in ill neonatal foals.[60,71] In those studies, foals with SIRS had significantly higher hospital mortality and lactate concentrations; moreover, hypoglycemia was associated with sepsis, positive blood culture, and SIRS.[60,71] Other studies have used SIRS as part of the criteria for inclusion to investigate sepsis.[61,69,74] In addition to the SIRS criteria noted earlier, one study also included other criteria, such as evidence of infection, cerebral ischemia or hypoxia, and trauma (fractured ribs, head trauma) as parameters that could fulfill the SIRS criteria.[60] Note that statistical association between SIRS and both mortality and lactate concentration were present only when the SIRS criteria included evidence of infection, ischemia, hypoxia, or trauma.[60] Other suggested criteria for severe systemic inflammation include scleral/mucosal injection (**Fig. 2**), petechiae, hemorrhage at the coronary band, and hypoglycemia (<2.2 mmol/L [<40 mg/dL]).[74]

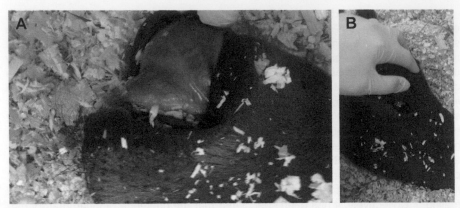

Fig. 2. A 3-day old thoroughbred foal showing clinical signs of vascular injection and hyperemia of the oral mucosa (*A*) and sclera (*B*) as a result of sepsis.

Collectively, use of the SIRS definition facilitated categorization of patients (ie, inclusion criteria for sepsis) and helped investigate associations between various blood parameters (eg, lactate) and systemic inflammation. In general, the SIRS definition in equine medicine may not only facilitate early clinical recognition of septic foals but also provide a better guide for inclusion criteria and cohort categorization for research studies. Although blood culture is considered essential by many clinicians to direct antimicrobial therapy in presumptively septic foals, reliance on positive blood culture alone to determine sepsis can lead to inaccurate and delayed results based on the sensitivity and specificity of blood cultures and the fact that foals may have received antimicrobials before blood collection. In addition, several days are typically needed to yield bacterial growth in culture. Alternatively, using a widely accepted SIRS definition in equine medicine may be superior to blood culture alone as a clinical method in identifying septic patients and/or identifying appropriate clinical candidates to be enrolled into prospective studies.

A widely accepted definition of SIRS in foals has not been established within the veterinary literature. Echoing the stated original purpose for the development of the SIRS criteria in people, the SIRS criteria in equine medicine should provide a conceptual and clinically practical framework to both define sepsis in the foal and establish an easy-to-apply set of clinical parameters that will facilitate stall-side detection of sepsis, thus allowing early therapeutic intervention.[1,3,8] In addition, these definitions should allow more uniformity of inclusion criteria for research studies involving foals. Based on these precepts, the definition (infection plus SIRS) and fundamental criteria for evaluating SIRS in foals remain similar to those of pediatric SIRS; namely, using the readily available age-specific vital (rectal temperature, heart rate, respiratory rate) and common clinicopathology parameters (complete blood count, blood gas analysis, lactate, glucose) to establish practical SIRS criteria (**Table 1**). For clinical purposes and ease of use, the authors propose 4 age groups, based on physiologic changes as the foal ages, for evaluating foals for SIRS: newborn (birth to 3 days of age), neonate (4–14 days of age), juvenile foal (15 days to 6 months of age), and weanling foal (7 months to 1 year).

The modified criteria for SIRS in children include the presence of at least 2 of the following 4 criteria, 1 of which must be abnormal temperature or leukocyte count: (1) core temperature more than or less than specific set temperatures; (2) tachycardia,

Table 1
Proposed SIRS criteria for foals, which require the presence of at least 3 of the following criteria, 1 of which must be abnormal temperature or leukocyte count

Parameter	Newborn Foal (Birth to 3 d of Age)	Neonatal Foal (4–14 d of Age)	Juvenile Foal (15 d to 6 mo)	Weanling Foal (7 mo to 1 y)
Fever or hypothermia (rectal temperature)	>102.6°F [39.2°C] or <99°F [37.2°C]	>102.6°F [39.2°C] or <99°F [37.2°C]	>102.6°F [39.2°C] or <99°F [37.2°C]	>102.6°F [39.2°C] or <99°F [37.2°C]
Tachycardia (beats/min)	>115	>120	>96	>60
Tachypnea (breaths/min)	>56	>56	>44	>20
Leukocytosis ($\times10^3$), leucopenia ($\times10^3$), or >5% band neutrophils[a]	>14.4 or <6.9	>12.5 or <4.0	>12.5 or <4.0	>12.5 or <4.0
Venous blood lactate level (mmol/L)	>5.0	>2.5	>2.5	>2.5
Venous blood glucose level (mg/dL)	<50	<50	<50	<50

[a] Varies with individual clinicopathology laboratories.

as defined as a heart rate of greater than 2 standard deviations (SD) greater than the normal for age in the absence of external or painful stimulus; (3) respiratory rate more than 2 SD greater than normal for age; and (4) leukocyte count increased or depressed for age or greater than 5% immature neutrophils.[8] Similar to children, many disease processes in foals are associated with tachycardia and tachypnea. Moreover, assessment of these vital parameters can be confounded by some foals becoming anxious when restrained by people, resulting in increases in these parameters. Therefore, vital parameters collected for the purpose of evaluating a foal using SIRS criteria should be collected when the foal is resting quietly or has become calm during restraint, if

Table 2
Vital parameters and white cell counts in foals at various ages

Age	Heart Rate Healthy Foal (beats/min)	Tachycardia (beats/min)	Respiratory Rate Healthy Foal (breaths/min)	Tachypnea (breaths/min)	WBC Healthy Foal (×10³ cells/µL)
Birth	104 ± 16	>136	71 ± 6	>83	6.9–14.4
1 h	97 ± 17	>131	40 ± 3	>46	6.9–14.4
2 h	75 ± 11	>97	—	—	6.9–14.4
4 h	84 ± 17	>118	57 ± 6	>69	6.9–14.4
12 h	87 ± 12	>111	32 ± 5	>42	6.9–14.4
24 h	91 ± 15	>121	42 ± 4	>50	4.9–11.7
2 d	96 ± 4	>104	44 ± 7	>58	—
3 d	90 ± 6	>102	44 ± 1	>46	5.1–10.1
4 d	94 ± 4	>102	46 ± 4	>54	—
5 d	102 ± 6	>114	—	—	—
6 d	100 ± 12	>124	—	—	—
7 d	88 ± 27	>142	42 ± 5	>52	6.3–13.6
8 d	86 ± 14	>114	—	—	—
14 d	83 ± 19	>121	38 ± 11	>60	5.2–11.9
20–22 d	84 ± 10	>104	38 ± 10	>58	5.3–12.2
28 d	77 ± 12	>101	34 ± 11	>56	5.4–12.4
41–43 d	76 ± 11	>98	—	—	—
8 wk	70 ± 13	>96	32 ± 8	>48	5.4–13.5
12 wk	69 ± 13	>95	27 ± 6	>39	6.7–16.8
4 mo	82 ± 8	>98	—	—	6.2–14.2
5 mo	88 ± 6	>100	—	—	6.4–14.6
6 mo	67 ± 7	>81	16 ± 2	>20	7.8–11.6
7 mo	57 ± 4	>65	—	—	—
9 mo	54 ± 1	>56	15 ± 4	>23	6.3–11.1
10 mo	57 ± 3	>63	—	—	—
11 mo	53 ± 2	>57	—	—	—
1 y	42 ± 1	>44	13 ± 2	>17	6.5–11.8
Adult	47 ± 2	>51	—	—	5.4–14.3

The definitions of tachycardia and tachypnea are based on adding 2 SD to the mean value of each parameter at different ages.
Abbreviation: WBC, white blood cell count.
Data from Refs.[75–84]

possible. In addition, blood glucose and lactate levels have both been significantly associated with SIRS and sepsis; therefore, the authors propose that these parameters be included as criteria for equine SIRS.[60,71] The authors suggest that the SIRS definition in foals used for clinical purposes require 3 or more of the following parameters to be present, 1 of which must be abnormal temperature or leukocyte count, using age group–specific reference intervals (see **Table 1**). Alternatively, for research studies, investigators may consider using exact age-specific vital parameters to evaluate foals (**Table 2**), using the same criteria as noted earlier (at least 3 of 6 criteria present, 1 of which must be abnormal temperature or leukocyte count). Note that the vital parameters in **Table 1** were summarized from several different studies.[75–85]

SUMMARY

The SIRS concept was created to facilitate early identification and prompt therapy for septic patients as well as to allow more accurate comparisons of septic patients in research studies. The pathophysiology of SIRS and sepsis is highly complex and is not fully understood, especially in the foal, in which further research is needed to understand the basic physiologic and molecular changes that occur with equine SIRS and sepsis. At present, sepsis remains a common clinical entity with variable reported survival rates ranging from 46% to 65%, whereas one small study reported 100% mortality in foals with septic shock.[69,86,87] As in the human counterpart, prompt suspicion and/or recognition of equine sepsis allows implementation of appropriate therapy and likely improves odds of recovery.[1,3,8] Although positive blood culture results from septic foals aid in targeted antimicrobial therapy, the use of SIRS criteria in equine medicine might help facilitate earlier recognition of sepsis in the clinical setting and also better categorize ill foals in research studies. The authors thus suggest the use of 4 specific age groups (newborn, neonate, juvenile, weanling) and 3 of 6 criteria (rectal temperature, heart rate, respiratory rate, white cell count, blood lactate level, blood glucose level) be present for evaluating for the presence of SIRS in foals. Continued investigations into SIRS and sepsis in foals are clearly required. Moreover, the refinement of definitions of severe sepsis and septic shock in equine medicine might facilitate notable recognition and treatment of these conditions and allow more specific development of goal-directed therapeutic end points.

REFERENCES

1. Bone RC, Balk RA, Cerra FB, et al. Definitions for sepsis and organ failure and guidelines for the use of innovative therapies in sepsis. The AACP/SCCM Consensus Conference Committee. American College of Chest Physicians/Society of Critical Care Medicine. Chest 1992;101:1644–55.
2. Adib-Conquy M, Cavaillon JM. Compensatory anti-inflammatory response syndrome. Thromb Haemost 2009;101:36–47.
3. Levy MM, Fink MP, Marshall JC, et al. 2001 SCCM/ESICM/ACCP/ATS/SIS international sepsis definitions conference. Intensive Care Med 2003;29:530–8.
4. Balk RA. Systemic inflammatory response syndrome (SIRS): where did it come from and is it still relevant today. Virulence 2014;5:20–6.
5. Bone RC. Sir Isaac Newton, sepsis, SIRS and CARS. Crit Care Med 1996;24:1125–8.
6. Vincent JL. Dear SIRS, I'm sorry to say that I don't like you. Crit Care Med 1997;25:372–4.
7. Marshall JC. SIRS and MODS: what is their relevance to the science and practice of intensive care? Shock 2000;14:586–9.

8. Goldstein B, Giroir B, Randolph A, et al. International Pediatric Sepsis Consensus Conference: definitions for sepsis and organ dysfunction in pediatrics. Pediatr Crit Care Med 2005;6:2–8.
9. Zaritsky AL, Nadkarni VM, Hickey RW, et al, editors. Pediatric advanced life support provider manual. Dallas (TX): American Heart Association; 2002.
10. Wilkinson JD, Pollack MM, Glass NL, et al. Mortality associate with multiple organ system failure and sepsis in pediatric intensive care unit. J Pediatr 1987;111;324–8.
11. Leteurtre S, Martinot A, Duhamel A, et al. Development of a pediatric multiple organ dysfunction score: use of two strategies. Med Decis Making 1999;19:399–410.
12. Leteurte S, Martinon A, Duhamel A, et al. Validation of the Pediatric Logistic Organ Dysfunction (PELOD) score: prospective, observational, multicenter study. Lancet 2003;362:192.
13. Graciano AL, Balko JA, Rahn DS, et al. Development and validation of a Pediatric Multiple Organ Dysfunction Score (P-MODS). Crit Care Med 2001;29(Suppl):A176.
14. Bosmann M, Ware PA. The inflammatory response in sepsis. Trends Immunol 2013;34:129–36.
15. de Jong HK, van der Poll T, Wiersinga WJ. The systemic pro-inflammatory response in sepsis. J Innate Immun 2010;2:422–30.
16. Angus DC, van der Poll T. Severe sepsis and septic shock. N Engl J Med 2013; 369:840–51.
17. Fry DE. Sepsis, systemic inflammatory response, and multiple organ dysfunction: the mystery continues. Am Surg 2012;78:1–8.
18. Khan FA, Khan MF. Inflammation and acute phase response. Int J Appl Pharm Tech 2010;1:312–21.
19. Mark KS, Trickler WJ, Miller DW. Tumor necrosis factor-alpha induces cycloocygenase-2 expression and prostaglandin release in brain microvessel endothelial cells. J Pharmacol Exp Ther 2001;297:1051–8.
20. Barkhausen T, Krettek C, van Griensven M. L-selectin: adhesion, signaling and its importance in pathologic posttraumatic endotoxemia and non-septic inflammation. Exp Toxicol Pathol 2005;57:39–52.
21. Charo IF, Ransohoff RM. The many roles of chemokines and chemokine receptors in inflammation. N Engl J Med 2006;354:610–21.
22. Denk S, Perl M, Huber-Lang M. Damage- and pathogen-associated molecular patterns and alarmins: keys to sepsis? Eur Surg Res 2012;48:171–9.
23. Erridge C. Endogenous ligands of TLR2 and TLR4: agonists or assistants? J Leukoc Biol 2010;87:989–99.
24. Werners AH, Byrant CE. Pattern recognition receptors in equine endotoxaemia and sepsis. Equine Vet J 2012;44:490–8.
25. Manson J, Thiemermann C, Brohi K. Trauma alarmins as activators of damage-induced inflammation. Br J Surg 2010;99(Suppl 1):12–20.
26. Lord JM, Midwinter MJ, Chen YF, et al. The systemic immune response to trauma: an overview of pathophysiology and treatment. Lancet 2014;384:1455–65.
27. Lewis DH, Chan DL, Pinheiro D, et al. The immunopathology of sepsis: pathogen recognition, systemic inflammation, the compensatory anti-inflammatory response, and regulatory T cells. J Vet Intern Med 2012;26:457–82.
28. Kawasaki T, Kawai T. Toll-like receptor signaling pathways. Front Immunol 2014;5: 1–8.
29. Mackay I, Rosen FS. Advances in immunology: innate immunity. N Engl J Med 2000;343:338–44.
30. Lin Q, Li M, Fang D, et al. The essential roles of Toll-like receptor signaling pathways in sterile inflammatory diseases. Int Immunopharmacol 2011;11:1422–32.

31. Romagnani S. Development of Th1- or TH2-dominated immune responses: what about the polarizing signals? Int J Clin Lab Res 1996;26:83–98.
32. Gogos CA, Drosou E, Bassaris HP, et al. Pro- versus anti-inflammatory cytokine profile with severe sepsis: a marker for prognosis and future therapeutic options. J Infect Dis 2000;181:176–80.
33. Burton AB, Wagner B, Erb HN, et al. Serum interleukin-6 (IL-6) and IL-10 concentrations in normal and septic neonatal foals. Vet Immunol Immunopathol 2009; 132:122–8.
34. Lipinski B. Hydroxyl radical and its scavengers in health and disease. Oxid Med Cell Longev 2011;2011:809696.
35. Castellheim A, Brekke OL, Espevik T, et al. Innate immune responses to danger signals in systemic inflammatory response syndrome and sepsis. Scand J Immunol 2009;69:479–91.
36. Wort SJ, Evans TW. The role of the endothelium in modulating vascular control in sepsis and related conditions. Br Med Bull 1999;55:30–48.
37. Rittirsch D, Flierl MA, Ward PA. Harmful molecular mechanisms in sepsis. Nat Rev Immunol 2008;8:776–87.
38. Cavaillon J, Annane D. Compartmentalization of the inflammatory response in sepsis and SIRS. J Endotoxin Res 2006;12:1515–70.
39. O'Brien JM, Ali NA, Aberegg SK, et al. Sepsis. Am J Med 2007;120:1012–22.
40. Chu AJ. Tissue factor, blood coagulation, and beyond: an overview. Int J Inflamm 2011;2011:367284.
41. Sarangi PP, Lee HW, Kim M. Activated protein C action in inflammation. Br J Haematol 2010;148:817–33.
42. Frick IM, Bjorck L, Herwald H. The dual role of the contact system in bacterial infectious disease. Thromb Haemost 2007;98:497–502.
43. Ward PA. The dark side of C5a in sepsis. Nat Rev Immunol 2004;4:133–42.
44. Ward PA. The harmful role of C5a on innate immunity in sepsis. J Innate Immun 2010;2:439–45.
45. Moore JN, Vandenplas ML. Is it the systemic inflammatory response syndrome or endotoxemia in horses with colic. Vet Clin Equine 2014;30:337–51.
46. Andersson U, Tracey KJ. Reflex principles of immunological homeostasis. Annu Rev Immunol 2012;30:313–35.
47. Rosas-Ballina M, Olofsson PS, Ochani M, et al. Acetylcholine-synthesizing T cells relay neural signals in a vagus nerve circuit. Science 2011;334:98–101.
48. Flierl MA, Rittirsch D, Nadeau BA, et al. Phagocyte-derived catecholamines enhance acute inflammatory injury. Nature 2007;449:721–5.
49. Osuchowski MF, Welch K, Siddiqui J, et al. Circulating cytokine/inhibitor profiles reshape the understanding of the SIRS/CARS continuum in sepsis and predict mortality. J Immunol 2006;177:1967–74.
50. Seitz M, Loetscher P, Dewald B, et al. Interleukin-10 differentially regulates cytokine inhibitor and chemokine release from blood mononuclear cells and fibroblasts. Eur J Immunol 1996;25:1129–32.
51. Shubin NJ, Monaghan SF, Ayala A. Anti-inflammatory mechanisms of sepsis. Contrib Microbiol 2011;17:108–24.
52. Jaffer U, Wade RG, Gourlay T. Cytokines in the systemic inflammatory response syndrome: a review. HSR Proc Intensive Care Cardiovasc Anesth 2010;2:161–75.
53. Ward NS, Casserly B, Ayala A. The compensatory anti-inflammatory response syndrome (CARS) in critically ill patients. Clin Chest Med 2008;29:617–25.
54. Hackett ES, Lunn DP, Ferris RA, et al. Detection of bacteraemia and host response in healthy neonatal foals. Equine Vet J 2015;47:405–9.

55. Cohen ND. Causes of and farm management factors associated with disease and death in foals. J Am Vet Med Assoc 1994;204:1644–51.

56. Brewer BD, Koterba AM. Bacterial isolates and susceptibility patterns in foals in a neonatal intensive care unit. Compend Contin Educ 1990;12:1773–80.

57. Marsh PS, Palmer JE. Bacterial isolates from blood and their susceptibility patterns in critically ill foals: 543 cases (1991-1998). J Am Vet Med Assoc 2001;218:1608–10.

58. Russell CM, Axon JE, Begg AP. Blood culture isolates and antimicrobial sensitivities from 427 critically ill neonatal foals. Aust Vet J 2008;86:266–71.

59. Venkatesh M, Flores A, Luna RA, et al. Molecular microbiological methods in the diagnosis of neonatal sepsis. Expert Rev Anti Infect Ther 2010;8:1037–48.

60. Corley KT, Donaldson LL, Furr MO. Arterial lactate concentration, hospital survival, sepsis and SIRS in critically ill neonatal foals. Equine Vet J 2005;37:53–9.

61. Cotovio M, Monreal L, Armengou J, et al. Fibrin deposits and organ failure in newborn foals with severe septicemia. J Vet Intern Med 2008;22:1403–10.

62. Pusterla N, Magdesian G, Mapes S, et al. Expression of molecular markers in blood of neonatal foals with sepsis. Am J Vet Res 2006;67:1045–9.

63. Gold JR, Perkins GA, Erb HN, et al. Cytokine profiles of peripheral blood mononuclear cells isolated from septic and healthy neonatal foals. J Vet Intern Med 2007;21:482–8.

64. Castagnetti C, Mariella J, Pirrone A, et al. Expression of interleukin-1β, interleukin-8 and interferon-γ in blood samples obtained from healthy and sick neonatal foals. Am J Vet Res 2012;73:1418–27.

65. Wu RQ, Xu YX, Song XH, et al. Relationship between cytokine mRNA expression and organ damage following cecal ligation and puncture. World J Gastroenterol 2002;8:131–4.

66. Wagner B, Burton A, Ainsworth D. Interferon-gamma, interleukin-4 and interleukin-10 production by T helper cells reveals intact Th1 and regulatory TR2 cell activation and a delay of the Th2 cell response in equine neonates and foals. Vet Res 2010;41:47–60.

67. Perkins GA, Wagner B. The development of equine immunity: current knowledge on immunology in the young horse. Equine Vet J 2015;47:267–74.

68. Secor EJ, Matychak MB, Felippe MJ. Transfer of tumor necrosis factor-alpha via colostrum to foals. Vet Rec 2010;170:51–4.

69. Castagnetti C, Pirrone A, Mariella J, et al. Venous blood lactate evaluation in equine neonatal intensive care. Theriogenology 2010;73:343–57.

70. Furr MO. Systemic inflammatory response syndrome, sepsis, and antimicrobial therapy. Clin Tech Equine Prac 2003;2:3–8.

71. Hollis AR, Furr MO, Magdesian KG, et al. Blood glucose concentrations in critically ill neonatal foals. J Vet Intern Med 2008;22:1223–7.

72. Corley KT, Amoroso L, McKenzie HC, et al. Initial experience with norepinephrine in neonatal foals. J Vet Emerg Crit Care 2000;10:267–77.

73. McKenzie HC, Furr MO. Equine neonatal sepsis: the pathophysiology of severe inflammation and infection. Comp Cont Educ Pract Vet 2001;23:661–72.

74. Dallap-Schaer BL, Bentz AI, Boston RC, et al. Comparison of viscoelastic coagulation analysis and standard coagulation profiles in critically ill neonatal foals to outcome. J Vet Emerg Crit Care 2009;19:88–95.

75. Stewart JH, Rose RJ, Barko AM. Echocardiography in foals from birth to three months old. Equine Vet J 1984;16:332–41.

76. Nagel C, Erber R, Bergmaier C, et al. Cortisol and progestin release, heart rate and heart rate variability in the pregnant and postpartum mare, fetus and newborn foal. Theriogenology 2012;78:759–67.

77. Knych HK, Steffey EP, Mitchell MM, et al. Effects of age on the pharmacokinetics and selected pharmacodynamics of intravenously administered fentanyl in foals. Equine Vet J 2015;47:72–7.
78. Ayala I, Montes A, Bernal LJ, et al. Electrocardiographic values in Spanish-bred horses of different ages. Aust Vet J 1995;72:225–6.
79. Visser EK, van Reenen CG, van der Werf JTN, et al. Heart rate and heart rate variability during a novel object test and a handling test in young horses. Physiol Behav 2002;76:289–96.
80. Ohmura H, Hiraga A, Aida H, et al. Effects of initial handling and training on autonomic nervous function in young Thoroughbreds. Am J Vet Res 2002;63:1488–91.
81. Stewart JH, Rose RJ, Barko AM. Respiratory studies in foals from birth to seven days old. Equine Vet J 1984;16:323–8.
82. Lavoie JP, Madigan JE, Cullor JS, et al. Haemodynamic, pathological, haematological and behavioural changes during endotoxin infusion in equine neonates. Equine Vet J 1990;22:23–9.
83. Koterba AM, Wozniak JA, Kosch PC. Ventilatory and timing parameters in normal horses at rest up to age one year. Equine Vet J 1995;27:257–64.
84. Armengou L, Jose-Cunilleras E, Rios J, et al. Metabolic and endocrine profiles in sick neonatal foals are related to survival. J Vet Intern Med 2013;27:567–75.
85. Harvey JW. Normal hematologic values. In: Koterba AM, Drummond WH, Kosch PC, editors. Equine clinical neonatology. Philadelphia: Lea & Febiger; 1990. p. 561–70.
86. Borchers A, Wilkins PA, Marsh PM, et al. Association of admission L-lactate concentration in hospitalized equine neonates with presenting complaint, periparturient events, clinical diagnosis and outcome: a prospective multicenter study. Equine Vet J 2012;44(Suppl 41):57–63.
87. Hart KA, Barton MH, Ferguson DC, et al. Serum cortisol fraction in healthy and septic neonatal foals. J Vet Intern Med 2011;25:345–55.

Sepsis and Septic Shock in the Equine Neonate

Christopher Langdon Fielding, DVM[a],*, Kiragos Gary Magdesian, DVM[b]

KEYWORDS

- Antimicrobial • Hemodynamic support • Source control • Blood culture

KEY POINTS

- Equine neonatal sepsis is associated with an increased mortality rate compared with other medical conditions affecting newborn foals.
- As sepsis progresses to severe sepsis and septic shock, the prognosis becomes worse.
- Recognition of sepsis in foals is poor given current laboratory and examination parameters.
- Early and aggressive treatment of presumed cases of neonatal sepsis is warranted.

INTRODUCTION

Sepsis and specifically the development of septic shock represent one of the most significant causes of morbidity and mortality in equine neonates. Although understanding of the pathophysiology of sepsis continues to evolve, the condition remains challenging to manage and failure is common despite considerable advancements in treatment. Early recognition of sepsis is essential to successful management and requires a coordinated effort between stable managers, field veterinarians, and neonatal intensive care unit clinicians.

This article reviews the recognition of sepsis/septic shock and current treatment recommendations for this condition. The research available on equine neonatal sepsis (ENS) is limited, but new information is available each year. This article brings together equine-specific information and incorporates the most recent human Surviving Sepsis guidelines that were published in 2012.[1]

Briefly, sepsis is defined in a patient in which the systemic inflammatory response syndrome (SIRS) is caused by infection (**Box 1**). In human critical care, SIRS includes alterations in two of the following parameters: body temperature, heart rate,

The authors have nothing to disclose or any conflicts of interest.
[a] Loomis Basin Equine Medical Center, 2973 Penryn Road, Penryn, CA 95663, USA;
[b] Department of Medicine and Epidemiology, School of Veterinary Medicine, University of California, Davis, 2108 Tupper Hall, Davis, CA 95616, USA
* Corresponding author.
E-mail address: langdonfielding@yahoo.com

Box 1
Definitions of sepsis, severe sepsis, and septic shock

Sepsis: The presence of a probable or documented infection together with systemic manifestations of infection

Severe sepsis: Sepsis plus sepsis-induced organ dysfunction or tissue hypoperfusion

Septic shock: Sepsis-induced hypotension persisting despite adequate fluid resuscitation

---

respiratory function, and peripheral white cell counts. This definition has been extrapolated for use in foals. Severe sepsis is a progression to the point that sepsis is associated with organ dysfunction, hypotension, and/or hypoperfusion. Septic shock is defined as sepsis-induced hypotension despite adequate fluid resuscitation, or vasopressor-dependent sepsis.

PATIENT EVALUATION

Early recognition of ENS is critical for early initiation of treatment, improvement in outcomes, but also for determining a realistic prognosis. Neonates may present for intensive care for a variety of conditions (eg, hypoxic ischemic encephalopathy, ruptured bladder) that may have a better prognosis than sepsis. Given that the mortality rate for ENS is as high as 50%, its recognition is important when discussing prognosis with owners.[2] In general, suspicion of ENS can be divided into three categories: (1) historical information, (2) physical examination, and (3) laboratory markers.

Although the criteria for the diagnosis of sepsis do not often include historical information, sepsis should be considered in patients that have specific historical events that serve as risk factors (**Box 2**). Historical information that would increase the index of suspicion for ENS include factors that existed before foaling, specific events that occurred during foaling, and developments in the period following foaling.

Owners and veterinarians may observe abnormalities in the mare before foaling that are cause for concern. These include premature lactation, increased vaginal discharge, or early signs of parturition. Although these findings are not uniquely associated with ENS, they warrant further evaluation and more intensive fetal monitoring, such as fetoplacental ultrasound or fetal electrocardiography. When evaluating an equine neonate, these prefoaling historical findings may cause the clinician to initiate treatment of ENS sooner than for a foal without these risk factors.

Prolonged second stage of labor is an important finding during foaling that may increase the risk for the development of ENS. Other concerning abnormalities might include an abnormal appearance of the placenta or the amniotic/allantoic fluids. Similar to prefoaling events, abnormal developments during foaling do not define

---

Box 2
Historical factors raising suspicion for sepsis

1. Historical factors before foaling: premature lactation, increased vaginal discharge, early signs of parturition

2. Historical factors observed during foaling: prolonged second stage of labor, abnormal appearance of fetal fluids, meconium aspiration

3. Historical factors following foaling: prolonged time to stand or nurse, abnormal behavior, failure of passive transfer

---

the septic neonate, but they should be part of the historical profile that helps to determine the likelihood of sepsis.

Developments following parturition are perhaps the most relevant historical events when identifying ENS. The time for the foal to stand and/or nurse may be prolonged in foals that are at risk for developing ENS. Likewise, any other abnormal behaviors or an overly "quiet" demeanor may be cause for concern. Most importantly, decreases in nursing frequency or activity level over time are strong indicators that sepsis could be present.

The veterinarian's physical examination of the equine neonate is the most readily available tool for the recognition of sepsis (**Box 3**). Abnormalities may include subtle changes in perfusion parameters or a very specific recognition of a septic focus (ie, swollen joint, enlarged umbilicus). The presence of petechiation of mucous membranes or skin of the inner pinnae and injection of mucous membranes should also raise the suspicion for sepsis; however these are not specific findings (**Figs. 1** and **2**). Unfortunately, physical examination parameters can be subjective and are often highly dependent on individual experience.

In a recent study that evaluated a large number of parameters for an association with sepsis, not a single physical examination parameter was included in the univariable or multivariable analysis.[3] This study did not include localizing signs of infection (eg, septic joints) as part of the analysis because these were included in the definition of sepsis. Given these disappointing findings, the search for early diagnostic criteria for sepsis continues.

Laboratory findings that are often part of the definition of sepsis include changes in white cell count and/or neutrophil count. However, increased creatinine, increased potassium, and decreased lymphocyte concentration were each associated with ENS in a multivariable model.[3] In addition, many studies have shown an association with IgG values either less than 400 or less than 800 mg/dL.[4,5] These are all common laboratory parameters that are obtained at initial evaluation of a sick foal and should raise the index of suspicion of sepsis (**Box 4**). Other studies have identified associations between sepsis and glucose or other parameters, such as lactate.[6,7] However most of these studies evaluate single variables (ie, blood glucose) and therefore have less ability to compare variables than a multivariable study.

When considering laboratory parameters associated with sepsis, it is important to distinguish between variables used to predict the presence of sepsis and those with prognostic value for survival. Multiple studies have shown the prognostic value of a variety of factors including blood glucose and lactate concentrations, and many others.[6–8] However, these parameters may be abnormal in sick foals with other conditions and are not necessarily specific to sepsis. Useful prognostic variables are helpful in predicting foal survival, but not necessarily for identifying ENS. One of the challenges in identifying specific markers of sepsis is the lack of consensus definitions

---

Box 3
Physical examination parameters that may be associated with sepsis/septic shock

1. Localizing signs of infection: enlarged umbilicus, swollen joint, wound with drainage

2. Signs of sepsis: Petechiae on the mucous membranes or within the pinnae of ears

3. Signs of hypoperfusion: decreased mentation, decreased pulse quality, increased heart rate (variable in foals), cold extremities, pale mucous membranes, increased capillary refill time, prolonged jugular refill, decreased urine output

4. Behavioral changes: decreased nursing frequency, increased periods of recumbency

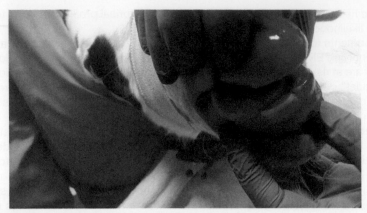

Fig. 1. Injected and hyperemic membranes in a septic foal.

of sepsis among studies. Some use blood culture results, whereas others use a combination of factors.

Sepsis-specific biomarkers have become a recent focus of research in foals and other species. A biomarker is "any substance, structure, or process that can be measured in the body or its products and influences or predicts the incidence of outcome or disease."[9] Biomarkers potentially represent a way to more accurately and efficiently diagnose sepsis. Unfortunately many of the options are not yet practical for use in a clinical setting because of either cost or availability.

In human neonates, biomarkers that have shown potential for identifying sepsis include C-reactive protein, procalcitonin, mannose-binding lectin, interleukin-6, adrenomedullin, triggering receptor expressed on myeloid cells-1, lipopolysaccharide-binding protein, serum amyloid A, and urokinase plasminogen activator receptor.[10] However, there is no consensus about the ideal biomarker for diagnosis of neonatal sepsis in humans. It is likely that the ideal biomarkers for sepsis identification vary among species and age groups.

In foals, sepsis biomarkers that have been evaluated include interleukin-1β, C-reactive protein, haptoglobin, and serum amyloid A.[11–13] Results of these studies have been disappointing and have not demonstrated these biomarkers to provide strong

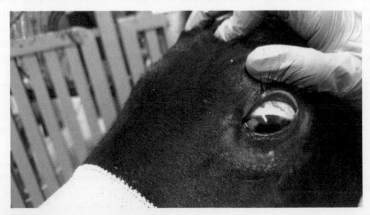

Fig. 2. Scleral injection in a septic foal.

Box 4
Factors associated with sepsis in foals in a multivariable analysis
Age (days)
Creatinine (mg/dL)
Lymphocyte count (cells/μL)
Potassium (mEq/L)
IgG less than 800 (mg/dL)
Data from Weber EJ, Sanchez LC, Giguère S. Re-evaluation of the sepsis score in equine neonates. Equine Vet J 2015;47:275–8.

or specific evidence of sepsis. **Table 1** lists some of the biomarkers that have been evaluated in foals with sepsis. Any new potential biomarkers should be evaluated as part of large, multivariable models to determine their usefulness in the identification of sepsis.

In summary, a combination of physical examination findings and laboratory data is required for a tentative diagnosis of sepsis while more definitive testing (blood or body fluid cultures) is pending. However, except for signs of local infection (swollen joints, umbilicus, and so forth), physical examination parameters are not specific or early indicators of sepsis. Routine laboratory variables may be useful for suspecting sepsis in foals; however, these test results may be altered with a variety of clinical conditions. New biomarkers are a promising area of research, but have not yet been shown to be valuable in diagnosing ENS. Given the limitations in the early, sensitive, and specific diagnosis of sepsis, early and aggressive treatment of at-risk foals is the most appropriate strategy while culture results are pending.

SEPSIS TREATMENT

Treatment options for sepsis/septic shock are divided into three main categories: (1) anti-infective therapy, (2) hemodynamic supportive therapies, (3) other supportive therapies.

Anti-infective Therapy

Anti-infectives are the cornerstone pharmacologic treatment of sepsis. In most cases of ENS, the offending organism is not known at the initiation of treatment, but bacterial organisms are the most likely associated agents with sepsis. Therefore, the early initiation of an aggressive, broad-spectrum antimicrobial protocol is warranted in cases of suspected ENS.

Antimicrobials should be started as soon as possible after evaluation and diagnosis of presumed sepsis. The topic of timing for antimicrobial administration has recently

Table 1	
Biomarkers that have been evaluated for identifying sepsis in equine neonates	
Biomarker	**Summary**
Serum amyloid A[12]	>100 mg/L highly suggestive of infection in young foals
Interleukin-1β[11]	Foals with sepsis had higher interleukin-1β than did healthy foals
Plasma C-reactive protein[13]	Not a useful biomarker for sepsis in foals
Haptoglobin[13]	Not a useful biomarker for sepsis in foals

received increased attention in human critical care. Several small studies have suggested that a delay (>3 hours) in the administration of antibiotics to patients with sepsis/septic shock can lead to increased morbidity and mortality.[14,15] However, a recent meta-analysis was unable to find a benefit from early antibiotic administration.[16] A large, prospective clinical trial would be ideal to answer this question, but until more information is available, early administration of antibiotics to foals with suspected sepsis is prudent. The Surviving Sepsis guidelines that were published in 2012 recommend administration of antimicrobials within the first hour following recognition of severe sepsis or septic shock.[1]

Equine ambulatory veterinarians can play a significant role in this treatment because they often evaluate foals earlier in the course of disease than do referral centers. By initiating antimicrobial treatment at the farm before transport, outcome from disease will likely be improved. **Table 2** outlines common antimicrobial treatment combinations, some of which can be easily started in the field. If renal function is unknown, one of the protocols that is safer for renal function should be used.

In a hospital setting, antimicrobials can be administered as intermittent infusions (typically two to four times per day) or as a continuous rate infusion (CRI). CRIs may be theoretically advantageous because they maintain antimicrobial plasma levels above the minimum inhibitory concentration for the duration of the infusion. Several small human studies have identified benefits when antibiotics are administered as a CRI as opposed to an intermittent bolus infusion.[17,18] However, larger scale

Table 2
Antimicrobials that can be used at initial evaluation of suspected ENS

Antimicrobial	Dosing	Notes
Amikacin	20–30 mg/kg IV or IM q 24 h Therapeutic drug monitoring recommended	Careful of aminoglycosides in foals with altered renal function; aminoglycosides typically combined with an antimicrobial with gram-positive spectrum
Ampicillin	20 mg/kg IV (or IM) q 6 h	Used in combination with an aminoglycoside
Cefotaxime	40 mg/kg IV q 6 h	Should only be used for foals with infections that are resistant to more commonly used antibiotics
Ceftazidime	40–50 mg/kg IV q 6 h	Should only be used for foals with infections that are resistant to more commonly used antibiotics
Ceftiofur	5–10 mg/kg IV or IM or SQ q 6–12 h	Can be used alone or in combination with an aminoglycoside
Gentamicin	8–15 mg/kg IV or IM q 24 h Therapeutic drug monitoring recommended	Careful of aminoglycosides in foals with altered renal function; aminoglycosides typically combined with an antimicrobial with better gram-positive spectrum
Metronidazole	10 mg/kg PO, IV or per rectum q 12 h	Used most commonly in neonates for enteric clostridial infections
Potassium penicillin	22,000 units/kg IV q 6 h	Used in combination with an aminoglycoside

Abbreviations: IM, intramuscular; IV, intravenous; PO, by mouth; SQ, subcutaneously.

prospective, randomized trials are ongoing and those results are needed to determine if there is a survival benefit to this practice.

Antimicrobial CRIs are suited to time-dependent antimicrobials, such as penicillins or cephalosporins. Concentration-dependent antibiotics, such as aminoglycosides, would not be appropriate for this method of delivery. The pharmacokinetics of ceftiofur and cefotaxime in foals have been published.[19,20] The authors have used ceftiofur, cefotaxime, ceftazidime, potassium penicillin, and ampicillin as CRIs. Generally the same total daily dose is used as for intermittent administration; the total daily dose is divided by 24 and then this dose is administered hourly by pump as a CRI. The antibiotic is often diluted in saline but care must be taken to follow any guidelines about compatibility, diluents, or storage. In addition, duration of stability at room temperature must be considered. **Table 3** outlines dosing protocols for some of the antimicrobials that can be used as CRIs for the treatment of ENS.

Blood cultures with antimicrobial susceptibility testing are an important component of the diagnosis of sepsis and can guide the choice of antimicrobials once available. However, their sensitivity, as compared with pathology results, suggests that blood culture cannot be used as the only basis for the diagnosis of sepsis.[21] Blood cultures are ideally obtained before the start of antimicrobial treatment, but delays in treatment initiation should be avoided. In humans, it is recommended that antimicrobials should not be delayed more than 45 minutes to wait for blood culture testing.

In summary, antimicrobial therapy should be initiated early in the course of disease and should include a broad-spectrum approach to therapy. A CRI can be used in particularly sick foals if this option is available. Antimicrobial therapy should not be delayed more than 45 minutes if blood cultures are to be obtained before starting therapy.

Hemodynamic Support

In addition to antimicrobials, hemodynamic support is considered the second major component of ENS treatment. The primary aspect of hemodynamic support is the use of intravenous fluids. Intravenous fluid support is important for initial replacement of deficits and for ongoing maintenance particularly in foals that do not tolerate oral fluids/nutrition. The topic of intravenous fluid administration in foals is extensive, but there are some general guidelines for the equine neonate with sepsis. Most fluid plans have three main components: (1) fluid type, (2) fluid rate of administration, and (3) end point to fluid therapy.

Table 3
CRI dosing for antimicrobial treatment of ENS

Antimicrobial	Dosing	Notes
Cefotaxime	6.7 mg/kg/h IV CRI, after loading dose of 40 mg/kg	Should only be used for foals with infections that are resistant to more commonly used antibiotics
Ceftazidime	6.7 mg/kg/h IV CRI, after loading dose of 40 mg/kg	Should only be used for foals with infections that are resistant to more commonly used antibiotics
Ceftiofur	0.17–1.6 mg/kg/h IV CRI, after loading dose of 5 mg/kg IV	Can be used alone or in combination with an aminoglycoside
Potassium penicillin	3600–4000 IU/kg/h IV CRI after loading dose of 22,000 IU/kg	Used in combination with an aminoglycoside

Abbreviation: IV, intravenous.

A balanced isotonic crystalloid is an appropriate fluid for initial resuscitation. There continues to be an ongoing debate about the role of synthetic colloids in fluid resuscitation; however, the lack of demonstrable benefit and the potential negative effects suggest that these fluids should be avoided at this time. Several approximately isotonic crystalloids are available (**Table 4**), with differing electrolyte composition. Given some of the recent evidence implicating the negative effects of hyperchloremia, relatively lower chloride fluids, such as Normosol-R (Hospira Inc., Lake Forest, IL) or PlasmaLyte A (Abbott Laboratories, North Chicago, IL), may be the most appropriate choice.

The authors use a typical protocol of 20 mL/kg bolus administration followed by reassessment. The duration of administration depends on the severity of hypovolemia and hypoperfusion, but can range from 5 to 30 minutes or longer. Boluses can be repeated, with each successive bolus usually being administered over longer duration, until perfusion parameters, such as urine output, extremity temperature, pulse quality, and blood lactate concentration, are improving. Signs of fluid overload, including pulmonary or tissue edema, should be avoided. Most equine neonates with suspected sepsis receive between 20 and 40 mL/kg of bolus fluid administration, although larger amounts may be necessary in very sick foals. However, given much of the recent evidence of the detrimental effects of fluid overload, larger amounts (>40 mL/kg) of bolus fluids should be administered with caution. If signs of hypoperfusion are still present after three of these 20 mL/kg boluses, then inotropes or vasopressors may be required.

In 2001, a landmark study by Rivers and colleagues[22] showed significant benefit in using a treatment strategy of early goal-directed therapy (EGDT) in critically ill human patients. This strategy used an early and aggressive fluid administration that achieved specific hemodynamic or perfusion targets, including central venous pressure (CVP), arterial blood pressure, and central venous oxygen saturation. For over a decade this was considered the standard for treatment of sepsis. However, in the last year, two new, large clinical trials have demonstrated very different results.[23,24] Both of these prospective, multicenter trials found no clinical benefit for EGDT and an additional review cited the significant use of intensive care unit resources when implementing EGDT.[25] This debate is far from resolution, but it is less clear that very aggressive fluid therapy early in the course of the disease is necessarily beneficial.

Once perfusion parameters have normalized and the bolus administration of fluids is finished, foals with ENS are transitioned to a maintenance fluid plan. Initially foals may require higher than maintenance requirements, but they are gradually transitioned to maintenance needs (approximately 4–6 mL/kg/h), depending on renal function and other concurrent diseases. Once on maintenance rates, and depending on renal function and oral intake of fluids, this phase of fluid administration requires a fluid that is lower in sodium and higher in potassium to avoid hypernatremia. If no milk is administered enterally, the authors commonly use a 50:50 to 75:25 ratio of balanced electrolyte solution (eg, Normosol-R or PlasmaLyte A) and sterile water where each bag is run

Table 4 Three common crystalloids used for resuscitation in ENS					
Fluid	Na+ (Meq/L)	K+ (Meq/L)	Cl- (Meq/L)	Ca++ (Meq/L)	Mg++ (Meq/L)
Normosol R	140	5	98	0	3
Lactated Ringers Solution	130	4	109	3	0
0.9% Saline	154	0	154	0	0

off of a fluid pump at equal rates (ie, each one is run at 50% of the total fluid rate for the patient). It is important that the sterile water mix with the balanced fluid before entering the vein to avoid hemolysis. Additional potassium and dextrose are added to these fluids depending on the requirements of the patient.

Although fluid support is a major component for the treatment of sepsis/septic shock, there is growing evidence that fluid overload increases morbidity and mortality.[26] Frequent body weight measurements (one to four times per day) can help to identify fluid overload. Monitoring for peripheral edema or changes in respiratory function (increased respiratory rate or effort, decreases in oxygen saturation of hemoglobin, suggestive of pulmonary edema) can also be helpful. Serial measurements of CVP can also suggest fluid overload. A high normal CVP (10 cm H_2O) should warrant limiting fluid rates.

In foals with septic shock, intravenous fluid administration alone does not achieve adequate blood pressure to maintain perfusion. It is difficult to identify a specific mean arterial pressure that should be maintained to reliably provide adequate perfusion. In EGDT, a mean arterial pressure of 65 mm Hg or systolic arterial pressure of 90 mm Hg has been advocated. It is unlikely that these same values would be ideal for all equine neonates; newborn or premature foals often require much lower pressures to maintain tissue perfusion. Regardless of the measured parameter, there are foals in which fluid therapy alone will not maintain adequate perfusion and additional treatments are needed.

In a foal with adequate fluid replacement, inotrope and vasopressor agents can be added to improve cardiac output and blood pressure, respectively. These medications are used commonly in equine anesthesia to counteract the effects of the inhalational anesthetics. Evaluating research from many species, it is unclear whether the use of inotropes or vasopressors has a significant effect on outcome and specifically which agents are most likely to be beneficial.[27] Patients with a poor response to fluid resuscitation (ie, septic shock) are likely to have a poorer prognosis as compared with those that are fluid responsive.

Dosages of inotropes or vasopressors that have been used in neonatal foals are outlined in **Table 5**. The exact application of these recommendations to foals is unknown, but dobutamine is the authors' initial inotrope of choice and norepinephrine is their initial vasopressor of choice. When advanced hemodynamic monitoring (eg, cardiac output) is not performed, the order of initiation of hemodynamic support should always be intravenous fluids, then dobutamine, then norepinephrine. The administration of vasopressors before improvements in cardiac output with fluid volume and inotrope support can be counterproductive.

In summary, the administration of an isotonic crystalloid fluid with a balanced electrolyte concentration, including a chloride similar to that of normal equine plasma, should be started immediately at admission. Repeated 20 mL/kg bolus administration should be used with reassessment between each bolus and discontinuation once perfusion has improved or fluid overload begins to become evident. Inotrope or

Table 5	
Dosing of inotropes and vasopressors for neonatal foals	
Medication	**Dosing Range**
Dobutamine	3–10 µg/kg/min[29,30]
Norepinephrine	0.1–1.0 µg/kg/min[28–30]
Vasopressin	0.3–1.0 mU/kg/min[30]

vasopressor agents can be used in foals with septic shock (refractory to fluid support alone) but the clinical benefit on overall outcome is unknown.

Supportive Therapies

There are many additional supportive therapies that are required to maintain a patient with sepsis/septic shock. They address potential problems including nutrition, coagulation, metabolic derangements, and recumbency. Studies supporting the use of these treatments are often conflicting in human patients and there is even less evidence for their use in foals.

Plasma transfusions
The administration of hyperimmune plasma to critically ill foals is a common practice in equine neonatal intensive care. The plasma may be administered for a variety of reasons including for colloidal support, for improvement of serum IgG concentration, and for other components within plasma (eg, antithrombin). In one study, there was a survival benefit to administering antiendotoxin plasma to foals as compared with another commercial plasma product.[31]

Glucose control
The concept of tight glycemic control was introduced over a decade ago and the recommendations have undergone continued revision.[1] Currently the recommendation is to avoid hypoglycemia and maintain blood glucose below 180 mg/dL in human patients.[1] This seems to be a logical strategy to adopt for foals until further research is available. A retrospective study in foals demonstrated that hypoglycemia (<75.6 mg/dL), hyperglycemia (>180 mg/dL), and marked glucose variability were associated with increased mortality.[6] Based on these findings, and those in humans, a target blood glucose concentration of 80 to 180 mg/dL seems reasonable in foals.

Corticosteroid therapy
Equine neonates that stabilize with intravenous fluid support or the addition of inotropes/vasopressors are unlikely to need corticosteroid therapy. The Surviving Sepsis Campaign Guidelines recommend use of hydrocortisone in adult septic shock only if adequate fluid resuscitation and vasopressor therapy do not restore hemodynamic stability.[1] For pediatric sepsis, the suggestion for hydrocortisone replacement is even narrower, when fluid-refractory, catecholamine-resistant shock was present along with suspected or documented adrenal insufficiency.[1] If a given foal with septic shock does not normalize perfusion despite fluids and inotropes/vasopressors, then the use of low-dose (physiologic dose) corticosteroids could be considered, but is of unknown benefit to date and requires further study.[32]

Sodium bicarbonate therapy
In cases of lactic acidosis or respiratory acidosis, treatment with sodium bicarbonate is not indicated. In neonatal foals with inorganic acidosis, such as those with enteritis and relative hyperchloremia, bicarbonate therapy may be indicated.

Gastric ulcer prophylaxis
There is not significant evidence to suggest that routine ulcer prophylaxis in foals with ENS is warranted. A recent multicenter retrospective analysis suggested antiulcer prophylaxis was associated with an increased risk of diarrhea development in foals.[33] Specific signs of gastrointestinal abnormalities (colic, diarrhea, and so forth) warrant the initiation of ulcer prophylaxis because these foals are at increased risk. Foals intolerant of enteral feeding are additional candidates for ulcer prophylaxis.

Diuretics

Furosemide administration can be used in cases of fluid overload. It is unlikely to improve outcomes in renal failure, but can allow for emergency fluid management to prevent pulmonary or significant tissue edema when renal function is impaired.

Nutrition

Enteral nutrition should be used when tolerated. Conservative escalation of amounts fed should be performed as the milk or milk replacer is tolerated. In general, recumbent sick foals require approximately 50 kcal/kg/d.[34] Otherwise, intravenous nutritional support should be used. Initially, dextrose can be used at rates of 4 to 8 mg/kg/min, but if enteral feeding is not tolerated after 24 hours, amino acids should be added. Lipids are added to parenteral nutrition when used for longer term (>2–3 days) provision of nutrition.

Low-molecular-weight heparin

There is no evidence to support the routine use of low-molecular-weight heparin in equine neonates, but evidence in other species suggests that there may be some benefit during sepsis. Until further research is available, low-molecular-weight heparin should be considered an optional treatment of ENS, especially when hypercoagulability is suspected or documented.

Management of recumbency

Nursing care is a major component of the treatment of ENS. Foals must be bedded appropriately and if recumbent they must be frequently repositioned to avoid pressure sores. Care of urinary catheters, intravenous catheters, and feeding tubes cannot be emphasized enough. Ophthalmic and oral care is necessary, and physical therapy for limbs in recumbent foals.

SURGICAL TREATMENT OPTIONS

In addition to the institution of appropriate antimicrobial therapy, source control is one of the most important aspects of treatment of ENS. Source control refers to the (1) drainage of an infected abscess, (2) debridement of infected tissue, or (3) removal of a foreign body. In foals this can include such procedures as the resection of an infected umbilicus or drainage and lavage of infected material from a joint. Removal of infected tissue or fluid should always be performed if medically possible and safe for the patient.

Any infected fluid or tissue that is removed should be submitted for culture and susceptibility testing. A Gram stain of the fluid can be performed initially to help guide antimicrobial therapy until a culture is available. If infection is localized, antimicrobials need to be chosen that penetrate well into infected tissues.

SUMMARY/DISCUSSION

Equine clinicians should have a high index of suspicion for sepsis in any equine neonate with a history, examination parameters, or laboratory values consistent

---

Box 5
Initial approach to foal with ENS at field evaluation

1. Administer intravenous broad-spectrum antibiotics

2. Administer repeat boluses 20 mL/kg isotonic crystalloid until
   a. Lactate less than 4 mmol/L (if available)
   b. Perfusion parameters normalize
   c. Urine is produced

Box 6
Initial approach to foal with ENS at hospital admission

Complete within 3 hours of admission

1. Measure lactate level
2. Obtain blood culture before antibiotic admission
3. Administer intravenous broad-spectrum antibiotics
4. Administer repeat boluses 20 mL/kg isotonic crystalloid until
   a. Lactate less than 4 mmol/L
   b. Perfusion parameters normalize
   c. Urine is produced
   d. Additional fluids are not indicated

      i. Signs of fluid overload

      ii. CVP greater than 10 cm H_2O

5 Consider inotropes or vasopressors if fluids are not indicated but hypoperfusion persists

---

with ENS. An initial field approach to the patient with ENS is outlined in **Box 5**. An initial approach to a foal with ENS presenting to a veterinary hospital is outlined in **Box 6** and should include initial evaluation (examination and laboratory), blood or other fluid collection for culture, immediate antimicrobial administration, and intravenous fluid support. Any infected fluid or tissue should be removed if possible. Foals that do not normalize perfusion following intravenous fluid administration are candidates for more intensive treatment with inotropes or vasopressors; however, owners should be aware of the more guarded prognosis in patients requiring vasopressors.

REFERENCES

1. Dellinger RP, Levy MM, Rhodes A, et al. Surviving Sepsis Campaign: international guidelines for management of severe sepsis and septic shock. Crit Care Med 2012;2013(41):580–637.
2. Hurcombe SD, Toribio RE, Slovis N, et al. Blood arginine vasopressin, adrenocorticotropin hormone, and cortisol concentrations at admission in septic and critically ill foals and their association with survival. J Vet Intern Med 2008;22: 639–47.
3. Weber EJ, Sanchez LC, Giguère S. Re-evaluation of the sepsis score in equine neonates. Equine Vet J 2015;47:275–8.
4. Tyler-McGowan CM, Hodgson JL, Hodgson DR. Failure of passive transfer in foals: incidence and outcome on four studs in New South Wales. Aust Vet J 1997;75:56–9.
5. Robinson JA, Allen GK, Green EM, et al. A prospective study of septicaemia in colostrum-deprived foals. Equine Vet J 1993;25:214–9.
6. Hollis AR, Furr MO, Magdesian KG, et al. Blood glucose concentrations in critically ill neonatal foals. J Vet Intern Med 2008;22:1223–7.
7. Corley KT, Donaldson LL, Furr MO. Arterial lactate concentration, hospital survival, sepsis and SIRS in critically ill neonatal foals. Equine Vet J 2005; 37:53–9.
8. Wilkins PA, Sheahan BJ, Vander Werf KA, et al. Preliminary investigation of the area under the L-lactate concentration-time curve (LACArea) in critically ill equine neonates. J Vet Intern Med 2015;29:659–62.

9. World Health Organization (WHO), International Programme on Chemical Safety. Biomarkers in Risk Assessment: Validity and Validation, 2001. Available at: http://www.inchem.org/documents/ehc/ehc/ehc222.htm. Accessed October 9, 2015.

10. Bersani I, Auriti C, Ronchetti MP, et al. Use of early biomarkers in neonatal brain damage and sepsis: state of the art and future perspectives. Biomed Res Int 2015;2015:253520.

11. Castagnetti C, Mariella J, Pirrone A, et al. Expression of interleukin-1β, interleukin-8, and interferon-γ in blood samples obtained from healthy and sick neonatal foals. Am J Vet Res 2012;73:1418–27.

12. Stoneham SJ, Palmer L, Cash R, et al. Measurement of serum amyloid A in the neonatal foal using a latex agglutination immunoturbidimetric assay: determination of the normal range, variation with age and response to disease. Equine Vet J 2001;33:599–603.

13. Zabrecky KA, Slovis NM, Constable PD, et al. Plasma C-reactive protein and haptoglobin concentrations in critically ill neonatal foals. J Vet Intern Med 2015; 29:673–7.

14. Weiss SL, Fitzgerald JC, Balamuth F, et al. Delayed antimicrobial therapy increases mortality and organ dysfunction duration in pediatric sepsis. Crit Care Med 2014;42:2409–17.

15. Wisdom A, Eaton V, Gordon D, et al. INITIAT-E.D.: Impact of timing of INITIation of Antibiotic Therapy on mortality of patients presenting to an Emergency Department with sepsis. Emerg Med Australas 2015;27:196–201.

16. Sterling SA, Miller WR, Pryor J, et al. The impact of timing of antibiotics on outcomes in severe sepsis and septic shock: a systematic review and meta-analysis. Crit Care Med 2015;43(9):1907–15.

17. Chytra I, Stopan M, Benes J, et al. Clinical and microbiological efficacy of continuous versus intermittent application of meropenem in critically ill patients: a randomized open-label controlled trial. Crit Care 2012;16:R113.

18. Lorente L, Jiménez A, Martín MM, et al. Clinical cure of ventilator-associated pneumonia treated with piperacillin/tazobactam administered by continuous or intermittent infusion. Int J Antimicrob Agents 2009;33:464–8.

19. Hewson J, Johnson R, Arroyo LG, et al. Comparison of continuous infusion with intermittent bolus administration of cefotaxime on blood and cavity fluid drug concentrations in neonatal foals. J Vet Pharmacol Ther 2013;36:68–77.

20. Hall TL, Tell LA, Wetzlich SE, et al. Pharmacokinetics of ceftiofur sodium and ceftiofur crystalline free acid in neonatal foals. J Vet Pharmacol Ther 2011;34:403–9.

21. Wilson WD, Madigan JE. Comparison of bacteriologic culture of blood and necropsy specimens for determining the cause of foal septicemia: 47 cases (1978-1987). J Am Vet Med Assoc 1989;195:1759–63.

22. Rivers E, Nguyen B, Havstad S, et al. Early goal-directed therapy in the treatment of severe sepsis and septic shock. N Engl J Med 2001;345:1368–77.

23. ARISE Investigators, ANZICS Clinical Trials Group, Peake SL, et al. Goal-directed resuscitation for patients with early septic shock. N Engl J Med 2014;371: 1496–506.

24. ProCESS Investigators, Yealy DM, Kellum JA, et al. A randomized trial of protocol-based care for early septic shock. N Engl J Med 2014;370:1683–93.

25. Angus DC, Barnato AE, Bell D, et al. A systematic review and meta-analysis of early goal-directed therapy for septic shock: the ARISE, ProCESS and ProMISe Investigators. Intensive Care Med 2015;41(9):1549–60.

26. Kelm DJ, Perrin JT, Cartin-Ceba R, et al. Fluid overload in patients with severe sepsis and septic shock treated with early goal-directed therapy is associated

with increased acute need for fluid-related medical interventions and hospital death. Shock 2015;43:68–73.

27. Oba Y, Lone NA. Mortality benefit of vasopressor and inotropic agents in septic shock: a Bayesian network meta-analysis of randomized controlled trials. J Crit Care 2014;29:706–10.

28. Hollis AR, Ousey JC, Palmer L, et al. Effects of norepinephrine and combined norepinephrine and fenoldopam infusion on systemic hemodynamics and indices of renal function in normotensive neonatal foals. J Vet Intern Med 2008;22: 1210–5.

29. Hollis AR, Ousey JC, Palmer L, et al. Effects of norepinephrine and a combined norepinephrine and dobutamine infusion on systemic hemodynamics and indices of renal function in normotensive neonatal thoroughbred foals. J Vet Intern Med 2006;20:1437–42.

30. Valverde A, Giguère S, Sanchez LC, et al. Effects of dobutamine, norepinephrine, and vasopressin on cardiovascular function in anesthetized neonatal foals with induced hypotension. Am J Vet Res 2006;67:1730–7.

31. Peek SF, Semrad S, McGuirk SM, et al. Prognostic value of clinicopathologic variables obtained at admission and effect of antiendotoxin plasma on survival in septic and critically ill foals. J Vet Intern Med 2006;20:569–74.

32. Hart LA, Barton MH. Adrenocortical insufficiency in horses and foals. Vet Clin North Am Equine Pract 2011;27:19–34.

33. Furr M, Cohen ND, Axon JE, et al. Treatment with histamine-type 2 receptor antagonists and omeprazole increase the risk of diarrhea in neonatal foals treated with intensive care units. Equine Vet J Suppl 2012;41:80–6.

34. Jose-Cullineras E, Viu J, Corradini I, et al. Energy expenditure of critically ill neonatal foals. Equine Vet J Suppl 2012;41:48–51.

Diagnostic Imaging of the Lower Respiratory Tract in Neonatal Foals

Radiography and Computed Tomography

Kara M. Lascola, DVM, MS*, Stephen Joslyn, BSc, BVMS, MRCVS

KEYWORDS

- Equine • Respiratory • Diagnostic imaging • Radiography • Computed tomography

KEY POINTS

- Digital radiography plays an essential role in the diagnosis of respiratory disease in equine neonates, allowing for more rapid stall-side image acquisition and display.
- The increased sensitivity of computed tomography (CT) imaging provides superior information regarding the characterization of lung disease and in conjunction with quantitative CT analysis allows for more objective image interpretation.
- Patient artifacts of respiratory motion and atelectasis, as well as residual fetal fluid in foals younger than 24 hours of age, can impact accurate image interpretation.
- Interstitial and alveolar patterns are most commonly identified radiographically in neonatal foals. Interpretation of patterns aids in the characterization of respiratory disease but is not specific to the cause of disease and often correlates poorly with clinical severity, progression of disease, or response to treatment.

INTRODUCTION

Pulmonary disease is a significant contributor to patient morbidity and mortality among sick equine neonates.[1–5] Although primary lung disease, such as aspiration pneumonia, is common in neonatal foals, a large percentage of sick foals acquire pulmonary disease secondary to systemic conditions, such as sepsis or systemic inflammatory response syndrome, both common problems in hospitalized neonates.[1,5] Diagnosis and characterization of respiratory disease in neonatal foals can be challenging and may be further complicated in sick foals with other comorbidities. Overt clinical signs of respiratory disease, such as dyspnea, cough, or nasal discharge,

Department of Veterinary Clinical Medicine, University of Illinois College of Veterinary Medicine, 1008 West Hazelwood Drive, Urbana, IL 61802, USA
* Corresponding author.
E-mail address: klascola@illinois.edu

Vet Clin Equine 31 (2015) 497–514
http://dx.doi.org/10.1016/j.cveq.2015.08.003
0749-0739/15/$ – see front matter

are variable and may be subtle or absent.[4,6,7] The use of diagnostic imaging, such as radiography or computed tomography (CT), plays a critical role in the diagnosis of respiratory disease. Radiographic imaging of the lungs has been the mainstay for the diagnosis of respiratory disease in equine neonates. In contrast to adult horses, in neonatal foals the radiographic technology required for acquiring thoracic images of diagnostic quality is readily available to most private practitioners. The increased availability of advanced imaging modalities, such as CT at university or specialized referral practices, is promising in that it may allow for more accurate anatomic and morphologic characterization of pulmonary disease in select groups of foals.

RADIOGRAPHY

Traditional film-screen and digital radiography are available to most equine practitioners in referral and ambulatory-based practices. Digital radiography has substantial benefits over traditional film-screen radiography in terms of portability, acquisition time, image quality (eg, digital processing and postprocessing techniques), and the convenience of immediate onsite image display.[8] Digital radiography has become standard for many equine practitioners in the last decade because of the demand of ambulatory equine veterinarians to have radiographs immediately available for viewing at off-site locations (eg, stables, training facilities, and so forth). These considerations are also important for critically ill neonatal foals requiring thoracic radiographs as it is often necessary to perform radiography in the stall not only at off-site locations but also in large veterinary hospitals. Few veterinary publications describe optimal neonatal foal thoracic radiographic techniques. It is important to highlight some pitfalls that may lead to reduced radiographic image quality, unwarranted radiographic artifacts, or increased radiation exposure to personnel.

Radiographic Imaging Protocol

Despite the large dynamic range seen in digital radiography (ability to produce images from a wide range of exposure settings), image resolution and anatomic detail can still be adversely affected when incorrect exposures are used. During underexposure the reduced x-ray beam density or penetration must depend on extrapolation of data from the surrounding pixels. The image may seem to be of diagnostic quality through the use of the digital image filters, look-up tables, and manual windowing (contrast/brightness) adjustments; however, subtle radiographic findings and anatomic/pathologic detail can be missed. Conversely, with overexposure, the x-ray beam can oversaturate the detector elements leading to obscured margins or complete obliteration of some structures. Radiographic exposure settings should be matched to the size of the foal but typically involve ranges of 80 to 90 kVp and 5 to 10 mAs and with exposure times short enough to minimize respiratory motion. Given the size of the animal, and despite digital techniques that can reduce the effects of scatter radiation,[9] a grid with a ratio of 8 to 10:1 should be used.[7,10]

For many neonatal foals, images can be acquired without sedation and with appropriate manual restraint. In situations when sedation is necessary, selection of drugs with minimal potential for respiratory and cardiovascular side effects is important, particularly in sick neonatal foals with significant respiratory compromise. Benzodiazepines, such as midazolam (0.02–0.1 mg/kg intravenously [IV] or intramuscularly [IM]) or diazepam (0.02–0.1 mg/kg IV), with or without the addition of butorphanol (0.02–0.1 mg/kg IV or IM), are routinely used for noninvasive procedures, such as radiographic imaging.[11] Standard views described for imaging in neonatal foals include lateral (standing or recumbent) and ventrodorsal. For most neonatal foals, the entire thorax can be imaged with a single lateral view; however, larger breeds or older neonates may require 2 overlapping views to fully capture both the cranial and caudodorsal lung regions.

Standing lateral views offer the advantage of reduced atelectasis artifacts in the dependent lung but may not be feasible in foals that are very young, sick, or unable to stand for other reasons. The superimposition of the overlying muscles of the forelimb may also obscure the cranial lung field when in a standing position (**Fig. 1A**).[7] Pulling the front limb forward improves visualization but is typically not tolerated in the standing foal (**Fig. 1B**). Imaging foals in lateral recumbency offers the ability to manipulate the forelimbs to visualize the cranial lung field. Two standard lateral views will allow full inspection of each nondependent lung and, thus, provide the most information regarding localization of pathologic changes. This information is essential when foals are imaged in lateral recumbency because of the development of atelectasis in the dependent lung.[1,6,7,10] Lateral views have been described in healthy, sedated foals positioned in sternal recumbency and offer the advantage of improved ventilation for patients as compared with positioning in lateral recumbency, but atelectasis may still be present in the dependent lung fields.[12] Ventrodorsal projections of the lungs allow for some additional information on lateral severity using a single image. This view is performed with the foal positioned in dorsal recumbency and, thus, may not be well tolerated in nonsedated foals or in sick foals with respiratory compromise.

Horizontal beam radiography for a standing neonatal foal allows for inspection of both lung fields during the one exposure; however, information on the lateral severity is reduced, and radiographic detail for the hemithorax closest to the x-ray generator suffers from minor magnification blurring. Horizontal beam radiography is particularly useful when inspecting for pneumothorax or pleural effusion. The neonatal foal is placed in lateral recumbency, which allows for subtle pneumothorax to be detected in the nondependent hemithorax (**Fig. 2**) and pleural effusion to be detected in the dependent hemithorax. It is repeated in opposite lateral recumbency for the contralateral effect. At the authors' institution, horizontal beam radiography is routinely added to the standard thoracic radiography series of small animals when trauma is suspected.[13] There are increased radiation safety considerations when using horizontal beam techniques primarily involving subjects distant to the x-ray beam direction (eg, adjoining hospital rooms and potential personnel). Radiation safety regulations may restrict this practice to designated sites or prohibit the use all together.

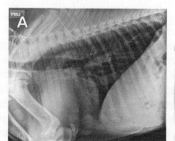 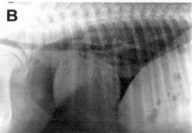

Fig. 1. A standing lateral horizontal beam thorax radiograph of a 5-day-old foal (*A*) and a laterally recumbent right lateral radiograph of a 4-day-old foal (*B*). Note the forelimb position and resulting superimposition with the cranial thorax in (*A*). Both radiographs show a mild amount of interstitial lung pattern in the caudoventral lung field consistent with atelectasis.

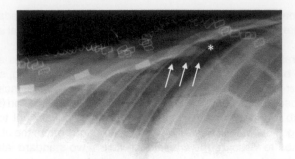

Fig. 2. A horizontal beam, ventrodorsal radiograph of a 1-day-old foal with history of postpartum trauma. The radiograph is highlighting the right lateral thoracic wall. Lacerations to the thoracic wall caused a small degree of pneumothorax (*asterisk*) and retraction of the lung lobe (*arrows*). The wound was recently repaired, and associated implants can be seen.

Radiographic Findings: Normal Foals and Artifacts

Normal neonatal thoracic radiographic appearance has been previously described.[7,10] Some unique features include a large thymus that fills the mediastinal space cranial to the heart and reaches a maximum volume at 2 months of age. The heart is also significantly larger in proportion to the thoracic cavity, when compared with the adult horse. The most significant normal thoracic radiographic findings are found in neonatal foals younger than 24 hours of age when there is a diffuse increase in lung opacity characterized as a prominent interstitial-to-alveolar pattern that obscures pulmonary vasculature and soft tissue margins. This increased opacity has been attributed to the combination of hypoinflation, residual fetal fluid in the airways, and the uptake of fluid into the interstitial space.[7,14] Given that early respiratory illness in neonatal foals will present with similar radiographic changes, the degree of affected lung can be underappreciated or completely masked by these normal findings.

Clearance of fetal pulmonary fluid from the alveoli and interstitium is expected to be complete within 2 to 6 hours after birth in several species.[15,16] Fluid clearance is primarily driven by active sodium absorption via airway epithelial sodium channels but is also influenced by increases in catecholamines, glucocorticoids, and alveolar Po_2.[17,18] The exact kinetics of fluid clearance in foals has not been described. Reports evaluating radiographic detection of fetal pulmonary fluid in healthy foals suggest that lung fields will appear clear by 4 to 12 hours after parturition.[10,14] Kutasi and colleagues[14] (2009) performed sequential radiographs in neonatal foals between 30 minutes of age and 48 hours of age and reported that resolution of lung opacity, and presumably clearance of fetal fluid, in the ventral lung precedes that of the dorsal lung. Discrepancies between timing of fluid clearance in these studies are most likely related to differences in study design, radiographic technique, and duration of recumbency (and thus amount of atelectasis) before image acquisition. It is not known to what extent the pattern and timing of clearance of fetal fluid may be altered or delayed in immature or sick neonatal foals with or without pulmonary disease; but Lamb and colleagues[10] (1990) reported that after 24 hours of age, radiographs should be able to aid in the differentiation of normal versus diseased lung.

Patient artifacts that may further complicate accurate interpretation of radiographic images include motion artifact from respiration and atelectasis. Respiratory motion artifacts appear radiographically as diffuse blurring of all structures. Imaging of foals at peak inspiration is ideal as it not only minimizes the impact of motion but also allows for better contrast between fully aerated lung and pathologic changes. Avoiding motion artifact is particularly challenging in neonatal foals with increased respiratory rates due to underlying disease.

Atelectasis is readily visualized in foals imaged in lateral or sternal recumbency[1,6,7,10,12] and is most likely due to compression (positional) atelectasis with or without concurrent absorption atelectasis. In a recumbent foal, particularly one on supplemental oxygen, atelectasis may develop over a short period of time. Positional changes will result in resolution of positional atelectasis within minutes.[7] The primary mechanism contributing to the development of positional atelectasis is compression of the dependent lung by overlying lung tissue. Cranial displacement of the diaphragm and increased pressure from abdominal contents may also contribute in specific cases when concurrent abdominal disease or uroperitoneum is present.[7] Neonatal foals may be predisposed to atelectasis as a result of immaturity in lung and chest wall compliance and possibly in surfactant.[19–21] Absorption atelectasis occurs in response to increases in inspired oxygen (F_iO_2).[22,23] This condition can occur with a F_iO_2 as low as 50% and, thus, may be applicable in sick foals administered supplemental oxygen before and during imaging.[24]

Interstitial and alveolar radiographic patterns may be visualized in atelectatic regions of lung. These patterns are not specific for atelectasis and may also occur in the presence of pneumonia (aspiration, viral, or bacterial) as well as other pulmonary diseases. In neonatal foals imaged in lateral recumbency, atelectasis has been characterized as a diffuse, mild to moderate interstitial pattern in the caudoventral lung region of the dependent lung.[7,10] The distribution may also be localized and asymmetric particularly in the perihilar regions.[7] In healthy, sedated neonatal foals imaged in sternal recumbency, atelectasis was characterized by an alveolar pattern that was most prominent in the caudoventral lung region with moderate interstitial changes noted primarily in the caudodorsal lung region.[12] The slight differences in characterization of atelectasis between these studies most likely reflects positional differences and the duration of recumbency but may also be influenced by the administration of IV sedation in foals positioned in sternal recumbency.

COMPUTED TOMOGRAPHY

Standard radiography plays an important role in the diagnosis and monitoring of foals with respiratory disease, particularly because of its relatively widespread availability and portability. However, in settings where both CT and radiographs are available, CT imaging may provide certain advantages over standard radiography. Current CT technology allows for rapid (within seconds), high-resolution, 3-dimensional, whole-lung imaging[25]; improves localization of disease; provides more accurate anatomic and morphologic characterization of all components of the lung (airways, vessels, parenchyma) and nonlung thoracic structures; is less impacted by respiratory movement or superimposition of overlying lung or other structures; and is better able to characterize nonspecific areas of consolidation.[26–29]

Previous limitations to the routine use of CT in veterinary medicine have included cost, time, preference for general anesthesia,[30] and availability. CT imaging is currently available at most veterinary teaching hospitals and select referral practices in North America. With current CT technology, the considerable reduction in time required for image acquisition has made this a more affordable and desirable diagnostic tool for hospitalized veterinary patients, particularly when short-term sedation can replace the need for general anesthesia in animals, such as sick neonatal foals with significant respiratory disease. CT imaging of the thorax has been well described in sick dogs and cats[31,32] and in healthy neonatal foals.[12,33] CT descriptions for sick foals include a case report describing a mediastinal mass in a 4-month-old foal,[34] sepsis in a neonatal foal,[30] and preliminary findings reported for a small number of critically ill neonatal foals.[35,36] CT imaging of the equine thorax is limited to foals or small ponies because of the fixed gantry diameter and table weight restrictions found with most CT systems in use in veterinary medicine (unless dedicated equine tables are used). Even with a gantry diameter large enough to accommodate an adult horse, the high exposure settings required to penetrate the torso, and reaching the detector panels, would involve photon energy levels that have little difference in attenuation by biological tissue, meaning there would be significantly less distinction between bone and soft tissue, with increased noise from scatter radiation.

Computed Tomography Imaging Protocol

As CT scanning involves ionizing x-ray radiation, patient preparation and scanning protocols are important to reduce the need for repetitive scanning and minimize radiation exposure to personnel. CT imaging in awake individuals is routine for humans and has been described for small dogs and cats using a specially designed restraint device.[37] For safety and practical reasons, neonatal foals cannot undergo imaging when awake. In the authors' personal experience, the administration of a single dose of midazolam (0.05–0.1 mg/kg) and butorphanol (0.05 mg/kg) is typically sufficient for CT imaging of spontaneously breathing healthy and sick neonatal foals and is well tolerated in.[33,35] In a limited number of healthy foals, additional sedation with a second dose of butorphanol and midazolam or the administration of propofol (1 mg/kg administered to effect) may be necessary to achieve effective sedation for imaging.[12,33]

Foals undergoing CT imaging of the thorax should be positioned in sternal recumbency with the head facing the CT gantry and the fore- and hind limbs extended cranially and caudally. CT findings in healthy, anesthetized neonatal foals positioned in dorsal recumbency have been reported with consideration to the appearance of atelectatic changes.[38] Interpretation of those images did not appear to differ significantly from foals imaged in sternal recumbency. The imaging technique described in healthy and sick foals includes a detail algorithm with the following settings: 140 kVp, 300 mA, 0.5-s rotation, 0.9 pitch, 0.9-s table speed, 512 × 512 matrix, 30-cm display field of view, 50-cm scan field of view, and 5-mm contiguous slice thickness reconstructed to 0.625 mm for the sagittal and dorsal reformations.[12,33] In healthy and sick neonatal foals, approximately 30 to 35 seconds are required to scan the entire thorax. At the authors' institution, the entire CT procedure, including sedation, transport to and from the stall, positioning of the foal, and scanning, typically requires 15 to 20 minutes, which is comparable with the time required for acquiring radiographic images.

CT allows for appreciation of the complex thoracic anatomy without any superimposition. CT also has the ability to distinguish each voxel in as much as 4096 shades of gray (Hounsfield units [HU]). This contrast resolution is superior to radiography, which is limited to only 5 opacities providing contrast resolution. With that being said, it is necessary to assess the entire thoracic CT series using multiple viewing windows of contrast and brightness levels. These windows should at least include a bone window (window length [WL]: ~300, window width [WW]: 1500), soft tissue window (WL: ~40, WW: 350), a lung window (WL: −500, WW: 1400), or optimized variations. The lung window will show the superior detail with contrast ranges covering the full spectrum of lung attenuation. This spectrum of attenuation includes gas pockets/bullae and hyperinflation/emphysematous lung at −1000 HU and less than −901 HU, respectively; normal lung at −501 to −900 HU; nonaerated lung at greater than −100; and collapsed, consolidated, or infiltrated lung at −100 to 100 HU.[27,33] Any tissue outside these ranges will appear completely white or completely black without any detail.

Computed Tomography Findings: Normal Neonatal Foals and Artifacts

In neonatal foals, normal aerated lung parenchyma will appear on CT as homogenous with soft tissue attenuating pulmonary vessels surrounding an associated bronchus (see **Fig. 2**). The vein should always be seen medial to the artery and bronchus. The pleural lining separating lung lobes can be normally visualized in feline and canine lung; however, the equine lung has no deep pleural fissures, so lung lobe distinction is based on anatomic regions of the bronchial tree rather than distinct interpleural boundaries. Reported findings attributable to atelectasis include a gradual and diffuse increase in lung attenuation (opacification) from dorsal to ventral within the lung parenchyma and interstitial and patchy to coalescing alveolar patterns with occasional air bronchograms identified ventrally and caudal to the heart in the areas of greatest attenuation (**Fig. 3**).[12,33] Subjective differences in the appearance of atelectasis are not identified between the right and left lungs of healthy foals; however, atelectasis may be more pronounced in neonatal foals 7 days of age or less when compared with those greater than 7 days of age.[33] Unfortunately descriptions of CT images in foals less than 24 hours of age have not been reported; thus, it is currently unknown what impact residual fetal fluid or hypoventilation may have on accurate CT image interpretation in very young foals.

Similar to radiography, there are artifacts that can arise from improper CT scanning protocols but also unavoidable patient-related factors. Patient artifacts that may impact accurate interpretation of CT images in foals are similar to those identified for radiography and include motion artifacts attributable to breathing and atelectasis. Motion is the most significant patient-related artifact experienced in veterinary imaging. In sedated, spontaneously breathing healthy foals, motion artifacts are typically minor but may become more pronounced in sedated, sick neonatal foals with significant respiratory compromise and associated tachypnea.

Motion artifact in CT appears as segmental blurring of the axial slices when the motion occurred and is typically most prominent at the widest point of the thorax (caudal lung fields). This blurring obscures sharp margins of thoracic structures (airways, ribs, pulmonary vasculature, and so forth) but can also apply a generalized increased

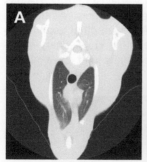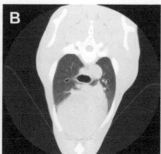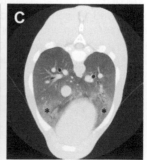

Fig. 3. Normal transverse CT images of a 5-day-old foal sedated and positioned in sternal recumbency. Image (*A*) is an image at the level of the cranial lung fields; image (*B*) is an image at the level of the carina and heart; image (*C*) is an image of the caudal lung fields. There is dependent/positional atelectasis noted in the caudoventral lung fields (*asterisks*). This foal is the same foal as **Fig. 1**A (CT: 5-mm slice thickness, detail reconstruction, WL: −500, WW: 1400).

interstitial lung pattern in the affected slices. If significant, the appearance can mask or even mimic pulmonary pathology, such as interstitial pneumonia. Strategies to control respiration, such as general anesthesia with controlled periods of apnea, may not be suitable for most critically ill neonatal foals. Some newer CT scanners are equipped with respiratory gating systems that synchronize the table movement with each breath cycle. These systems include bellows-belts that sense respiratory motion, cameras with movement tracking software, or spirometers that connect to an anesthetic breathing apparatus to detect changes in air pressure with each breathing cycle.

The mechanisms contributing to atelectasis in neonatal foals sedated for CT are most likely similar to those proposed for neonatal foals undergoing standard radiography but may be further influenced by the medications used for IV sedation and their potential impact on ventilation.[33] In healthy, sedated foals, scored comparisons between CT images and radiographs (obtained immediately following CT) revealed similar descriptive findings regarding the distribution of atelectasis for both modalities; but radiographic images were scored lower (ie, less severe) than CT images, suggesting a more pronounced appearance of atelectasis on CT images.[12] Alveolar recruitment maneuvers (ARMs) are often used in CT imaging in order to open atelectatic regions of lung and maximize lung aeration for improved contrast between normal aerated lung and areas of disease.[39–41] Evaluation of the use of single-breath manual ARMs of 10, 20, and 30 cm H_2O in anesthetized neonatal foals undergoing CT imaging has been performed.[38] Subjectively, manual ARMs did not eliminate atelectasis but resulted in minor reductions of atelectasis in the dependent lung and eliminated areas of increased attenuation in the nondependent lung, thus providing for a more homogenous appearance of lung attenuation.

Quantitative Computed Tomography Analysis

CT measures individual voxel densities (Hounsfield units) and displays the information for qualitative (subjective) assessment using axial slices of 2-dimensional spatial distributions, resliced into reconstructed planes (multiplanar reconstruction), or combined into 3-dimensional volume-rendered reconstructions (**Fig. 4**).[42] Subjective assessment of lung CT is not only difficult but also requires learned skill to detect and identify CT features, with occasional discrepancies between experienced radiologists. Quantitative analysis aims to provide automated, reproducible, and clinically useful diagnostic information from CT changes. It has been heavily explored in human lung imaging in the form of histogram analysis (HA), which plots voxel frequency against density. HA has been used in computer-aided diagnosis to evaluate disease severity, distribution, and progression and to monitor the response to therapy. Although other quantitative analysis techniques using regions of interest have been reported in veterinary medicine,[23,33,43,44] HA techniques have been published infrequently and have shown

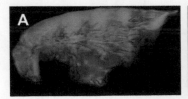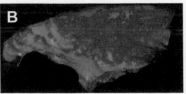

Fig. 4. CT volume-rendered reconstruction of the lungs of a normal 5-day-old foal (*A*) and a 6-day-old foal with severe bronchopneumonia (*B*). Blue represents normal lung with density ranges between −900 and −400 HU. Orange/red lung represents lung parenchyma with a density greater than −400 HU.

some challenges in accurately segmenting the entire lung field with exclusion of adjacent soft tissues that have similar densities to diseased lung.[12,33,45]

There are few quantitative lung CT techniques reported in neonatal foals.[12,35,38] These studies combined both semiautomated lung segmentation using density threshold limits with manual segmentation to include the full lung fields including dense atelectatic lung. This process is labor intensive and time consuming; each subject required approximately 45 to 90 minutes to complete (Lascola, Schliewert, personal communication, 2013). A manual technique used in ponies was estimated to take up to 8 hours to complete.[46] Reich and colleagues[46] (2014) also looked at shortening the segmentation process using an interpolation method of interspaced slices to calculate volume and overall lung density. However, this technique did not use a threshold segmentation tool, so they were unable to shorten the process to less than 1.5 hours. Their process was also unable to provide histogram analysis but instead gave an overall mean lung density and volume.

The authors have recently applied newer techniques that use multiple stages of automated segmentation to include the entire lung field regardless of the presence of atelectasis (**Fig. 5**), consolidation or infiltration, and with exclusion of nonpulmonary soft tissues.[35,38,47] This process takes less than 10 minutes and showed no significant differences in HA from those generated by the manual segmentation techniques. The authors are now collaborating on a fully automated equine neonatal segmentation program to shorten this time further. It is hoped that the HA research that this has facilitated in neonatal foals will provide more accurate information on respiratory disease severity and prognosis as well as augment treatment protocols. An example of HA created using these techniques can be seen in **Fig. 6**.

SUMMARY OF RADIOGRAPHIC FINDINGS IN NEONATAL FOALS WITH LOWER RESPIRATORY DISEASE

Radiography is useful for aiding in the diagnosis of a variety of lower respiratory disorders that are of concern to neonatal foals, including neonatal equine respiratory distress

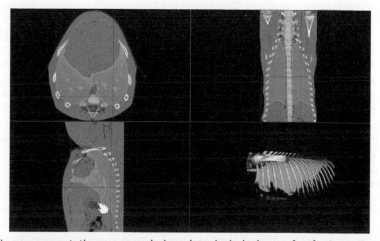

Fig. 5. Lung segmentation process designed to include lung of soft tissue density, yet exclude nonthoracic adjacent soft tissue yet. The gas within the stomach has been altered to a mineral density to help with the process. The lower right image shows the final volume-rendered image of the lung (*green*).

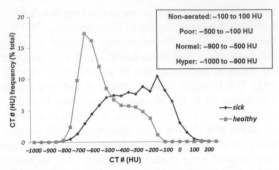

Fig. 6. Histogram lung density analysis of a healthy (*square plots*) and sick (*diamond plots*) neonatal foal created from lung segmentation. Note the trend for increased density toward the higher Hounsfield units for the sick foal and the peak of aerated lung tissue (−700 HU) for the healthy foal.

syndrome (NERDS), pneumonia (aspiration, bacterial, or viral), and equine neonatal acute lung injury (EqNALI) or equine acute respiratory distress syndrome (EqNARDS). Radiographic lung patterns seen in neonatal foals have been previously described[7,48] and have been extrapolated from adult horses and small animals. Radiographic patterns typically grouped into interstitial, nodular, alveolar, and bronchial may aid in the characterization of respiratory disease but are not specific to the cause of disease or location of the disease histologically, correlate poorly with clinical severity, and will lag behind progression or response to treatment. Furthermore, many changes can be due to artifacts from improper exposure settings or physiologic changes (eg, expiration causing an interstitial lung pattern, abdominal distension).[7,46] Radiographic findings will also change over the course of disease; thus, sequential imaging may be necessary to fully characterize the radiographic findings associated with respiratory disease and to best monitor patients for disease progression and resolution.

The appearance of an interstitial lung pattern comprises a hazy increase in opacity over the affected area. It leads to mild blurring of the pulmonary vasculature and airways becoming more prominent. The interstitial lung pattern can progress to form a reticulated pattern, which is due to infiltrating parenchymal bands of soft tissue (**Fig. 7**). A bronchial lung pattern is typically seen in conjunction with interstitial disease. The progressing and coalescing interstitial pattern tends to form peribronchial cuffing or rings of increased opacity. An uncomplicated bronchial lung pattern (bronchial wall mineralization) is uncommon in the neonatal foal. An alveolar lung pattern can develop on its own or as a progression of severe interstitial disease. It too can be regional or diffuse, but the increase in soft tissue opacity causes border effacement with surrounding soft tissue structures (eg, heart, caudal vena cava, pulmonary vasculature). If the airways are unaffected, then air bronchograms will be seen. The alveolar pattern implies complete collapse or consolidation. Nodular patterns in neonatal foals likely represent an artifactual concentration of interstitial lung pattern. Miliary nodules have been described in fetal lung infections with *Actinobacillus equuli*.[7]

In a review by Lester and Lester[7] (2001) describing radiographic findings in healthy, immature, and sick neonatal foals, the interstitial pattern was the most common radiographic pattern identified. Bedenice and colleagues (2003) retrospectively evaluated radiographs from 75 hospitalized neonatal foals with suspected respiratory disease. The most frequently identified pattern in this study was an interstitial-alveolar pattern, with primary alveolar disease most commonly identified in the caudoventral lung. The discrepancy between these reports in patterns may be attributable to differences in

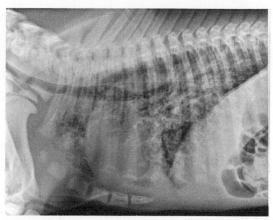

Fig. 7. Lateral radiograph (laterally recumbent) of a 2-day-old foal with a severe reticular interstitial lung pattern. Necropsy confirmed diffuse segmental interstitial pneumonia. Note a radiopaque feeding tube marker is seen within the esophagus.

the populations of foals evaluated, duration and type of recumbency before image acquisition, and potentially radiographic technique.

Both Lester and Lester[7] (2001) and Bedenice and colleagues (2003) reported the identification of radiographic changes most frequently in the caudodorsal lung with increased severity in this region corresponding to reduced survival of foals. Bedenice and colleagues[6] (2003) reported that combined caudodorsal and caudoventral involvement was found in most foals (63%). Involvement of the cranioventral lung seems to be the least common.[7] Furthermore, cranioventral pathology may only accompany concurrent caudodorsal and caudoventral pathology and may correspond to more severe clinical signs of respiratory disease.[1] When foals with sequential radiographs were evaluated, resolution of radiographic abnormalities typically progressed in a dorsal-to-ventral direction with the cranioventral lung clearing last. Both studies highlighted the challenges associated with the evaluation of the craniodorsal lung region due to the superimposition of soft tissue structures.

Radiographic findings in immature foals have been previously reviewed.[7,10] NERDS (previously referred to as respiratory distress syndrome or hyaline membrane disease) represents a distinct clinical syndrome of severe respiratory distress in foals less than 24 hours of age resulting from a primary surfactant deficiency.[5] These foals will present with severe radiographic changes that can be characterized as a severe, coalescing alveolar pattern distributed throughout all lung fields. Air bronchograms are often noted, and the cardiac silhouette and margins of the diaphragm are typically obscured.[4,5,7] Positive pressure ventilation with or without exogenous surfactant administration will result in at least temporary improvement in radiographic abnormalities.[5] Other respiratory diseases that may cause radiographic changes in foals less than 24 hours of age include meconium aspiration or EqNALI/EqNARDS secondary to sepsis.

Aspiration pneumonia occurs secondary to milk aspiration in neonatal foals with a poor suckle reflex or dysphagia secondary to weakness or perinatal asphyxia syndrome.[4] Radiographic imaging is useful for aiding in the diagnosis aspiration pneumonia, although clinical recognition of aspiration may be delayed in some foals. Radiographically, an alveolar pattern with or without associated air bronchograms is typically found in the caudoventral lung but may be localized to the perihilar region (**Fig. 8**).[4,7] Other causes of aspiration pneumonia may include aspiration of gastric

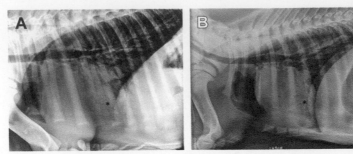

Fig. 8. A standing lateral radiograph of a 4-day-old foal (*A*) and a laterally recumbent radiograph of a 3-day-old foal (*B*), each with aspiration pneumonia (*asterisks*). The differences in forelimb superimposition can be clearly seen.

contents or perinatal aspiration of meconium (meconium aspiration syndrome). The sequelae of meconium aspiration may be more significant compared with aspiration of milk because of the potential for a chemical pneumonitis and mechanical obstruction caused by the meconium.[49] This syndrome is more common in human infants and is considered relatively rare in foals. Radiographic changes are more severe and diffusely distributed throughout the lung.

Radiographic findings associated with pneumonia secondary to viral infection or hematogenous spread of bacteria in foals with bacterial sepsis are typically diffusely distributed throughout the caudodorsal or entire lung.[1,4,7] Radiographic patterns may range from a diffuse interstitial pattern to a more severe diffuse and coalescing alveolar pattern (**Fig. 9**). Perinatal viral infection with agents, such as Equine Herpes Virus - 1 (EHV-1) or Equine Viral Arteritis (EVA), may occur rarely in neonatal foals and is associated with a severe, rapidly progressive and fatal interstitial pneumonia.[36,50,51] Radiographic findings are not well described for these foals most likely because of their rapid clinical demise.

Progression of primary pulmonary disease, bacterial sepsis, or perinatal viral disease to EqNALI or EqNARDS is a significant risk in sick neonates and carries a poorer prognosis. In humans, the standard diagnostic criteria for acute lung injury (ALI)/acute respiratory distress syndrome (ARDS) include the presence of bilateral pulmonary

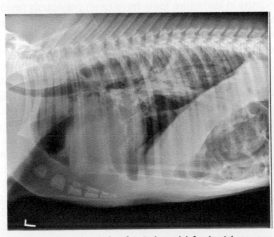

Fig. 9. A laterally recumbent radiograph of a 6-day-old foal with severe bronchointerstitial pneumonia.

infiltrates, noncardiogenic pulmonary edema, and severe hypoxemia as defined by a P_aO_2/F_iO_2 ratio of less than 200 mm Hg for ARDS and less than 300 mm Hg for ALI.[52] These criteria are similar for neonatal foals with modifications to account for potential age-related differences in gas exchange and allowance for bilateral or diffuse infiltrates to be identified on thoracic radiographs in more than one quadrant or lung lobe.[5] Radiographic findings of ALI/ARDS are best described for older foals but can be applied to neonatal foals and include a prominent, diffuse interstitial pattern with an overlying multifocal to diffuse coalescing alveolar pattern with air bronchograms.[36,53–55] The onset of ALI/ARDS is rapid; clinical signs during the early exudative phase may precede obvious radiographic abnormalities,[1] particularly if concurrent primary pulmonary disease is not present. Sequential radiographs may be useful to monitor not only disease progression but also resolution. Reports in older foals suggest relatively rapid resolution in radiographic abnormalities over several days in foals recovering from ARDS.[53]

Pneumothorax

Pneumothorax is a common cause of respiratory distress in neonatal foals, but the finding itself is relatively nonspecific and can be associated with other extensive changes to the lung parenchyma. It has been seen reported in cases of trauma associated with parturition (rib fractures and laceration of the pleura)[56–58] and secondary to sepsis (rupture bullae).[30] A small amount of pneumothorax, or pulmonary bullae, can be easily missed on ultrasound and standard radiography. In a standing lateral view, pneumothorax can be seen as gas opacity in the caudodorsal lung fields and associated with ventral collapse of the lung (increased in density). On lateral views, it may be difficult to appreciate, as it rises to the nondependent lateral thoracic wall where it becomes superimposed over the lung lobes. For these reasons, the authors recommend laterally recumbent horizontal beam radiography (see **Fig. 2**), or CT, to aid in the detection of small amounts of pneumothorax or clinically relevant pulmonary bulla (**Fig. 10**).

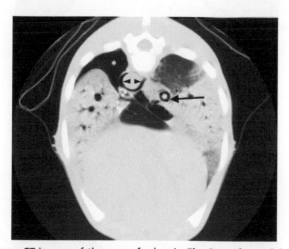

Fig. 10. A transverse CT image of the same foal as in **Fig. 9**, performed 1 day after radiography. There is diffuse consolidation of the right caudal lung lobe and portions of the left caudal lung lobe. There is a moderate degree of right-sided pneumothorax (*asterisk*), concurrent transecting perivenous emphysema (*arrow*), and pneumomediastinum surrounding the aorta (*arrowheads*) (CT: 5-mm slice thickness, detail reconstruction, WL: −500, WW: 1400).

Secondary changes that may accompany pneumothorax include rib fractures and pleural effusion (hemothorax). Detection of rib fractures may arise during the physical examination or during ultrasonography, which is considered more accurate then radiography, and become clearly visible with CT.[57]

SUMMARY OF COMPUTED TOMOGRAPHY FINDINGS IN NEONATAL FOALS WITH LOWER RESPIRATORY DISEASE

Descriptions of CT images of the lungs of neonatal foals are limited[30,35,36]; CT descriptive lung patterns for pathologic changes must, therefore, be extrapolated from small animal and human descriptive articles. Typical lung patterns include emphysematous, nodular, reticular, ground-glass, crazy-paving, and consolidation, to name a few.[59,60] Additional variations may also exist. Reported findings on CT of a neonatal foal with EqALI/EqARDS included a diffuse, bilateral, patchy to coalescing alveolar pattern with air bronchograms most pronounced in the ventral lungs that extended into the caudodorsal lungs.[36] The use of CT may be able to play a greater role in the diagnosis and characterization of EqNALI/EqNARDS. Its use is reported in small animals; in humans, CT has played a central role in understanding the pathophysiology of ARDS and is considered more accurate than chest radiography for detecting the underlying causes of and complications associated with ARDS.[61–63]

The authors have seen some neonatal respiratory cases through CT; in a few cases, the availability of both radiography and CT has allowed for comparisons between the two imaging modalities. When comparing the two modalities, the authors thought there was an underappreciation of pulmonary disease, characteristics, and distribution with radiography when compared with CT. Radiography of one neonatal foal with ARDS secondary to concurrent sepsis and aspiration pneumonia showed diffuse

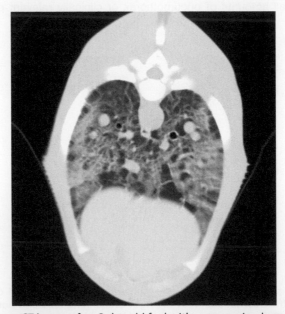

Fig. 11. A transverse CT image of an 8-day-old foal with crazy-paving lung pattern, showing extensive interlobular septal thickening surrounding both ground-glass interstitial pattern and emphysematous lung. Final diagnosis was ARDS secondary to septicemia (CT: 5-mm slice thickness, detail reconstruction, WL: −500, WW: 1400).

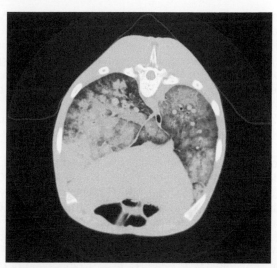

Fig. 12. A transverse CT image of a 6-day-old foal with diffuse bronchointerstitial lung pattern. It is characterized by diffuse interstitial ground-glass opacity to coalescing alveolar consolidation. Bronchial walls show diffuse, asymmetric wall thickening and narrowing. Final diagnosis was diffuse bronchopneumonia. This foal is the same foal as in **Fig. 4**B (CT: 5-mm slice thickness, detail reconstruction, WL: −500, WW: 1400).

reticular interstitial lung patterns but with relatively normal lung in the caudoventral lung fields. CT assessment, however, characterized this change as a crazy-paving lung pattern, showing extensive interlobular septal thickening surrounding both the interstitial pattern and emphysematous lung. Furthermore, the previously thought normal caudoventral lung fields were equally affected (**Fig. 11**).

A case of diffuse bronchopneumonia showed mixed distributions of multiple CT lung patterns. Diffuse interstitial or ground-glass opacity was seen throughout the lung fields, but patchy alveolar consolidation was seen asymmetrically in both dependent and nondependent lung. Bronchial lung pattern was also present and seen as 2 forms: bronchial wall thickening and peribronchial cuffing. This case highlighted both the myriad of lung changes that can be seen but also the severity and extent (**Fig. 12**). Foals with bronchopneumonia that survived had subjectively fewer unique lung patterns present, with less of the caudodorsal lung fields affected.

REFERENCES

1. Bedenice D, Heuwieser W, Solano M, et al. Risk factors and prognostic variables for survival of foals with radiographic evidence of pulmonary disease. J Vet Intern Med 2003;17(6):868–75.
2. Beech J. Respiratory problems in foals. Vet Clin North Am Equine Pract 1985; 1(1):131–49.
3. Freeman L, Paradis MR. Evaluating the effectiveness of equine neonatal care. Vet Med 1992;87:921–62. Available at: http://agris.fao.org/agris-search/search.do?recordID=US9306437. Accessed August 3, 2015.
4. Wilkins PA. Lower respiratory problems of the neonate. Vet Clin North Am Equine Pract 2003;19(1):19–33.
5. Wilkins PA, Otto CM, Baumgardner JE, et al. Acute lung injury and acute respiratory distress syndromes in veterinary medicine: consensus definitions: the Dorothy

Russell Havemeyer Working Group on ALI and ARDS in Veterinary Medicine. J Vet Emerg Crit Care 2007;17(4):333–9.

6. Bedenice D, Heuwieser W, Brawer R, et al. Clinical and prognostic significance of radiographic pattern, distribution, and severity of thoracic radiographic changes in neonatal foals. J Vet Intern Med 2003;17(6):876–86.

7. Lester GD, Lester NV. Abdominal and thoracic radiography in the neonate. Vet Clin North Am Equine Pract 2001;17(1):19–46, v.

8. Nelson NC, Zekas LJ, Reese DJ. Digital radiography for the equine practitioner: basic principles and recent advances. Vet Clin North Am Equine Pract 2012; 28(3):483–95.

9. Lo WY, Hornof WJ, Zwingenberger AL, et al. Multiscale image processing and antiscatter grids in digital radiography. Vet Radiol Ultrasound 2009;50(6):569–76.

10. Lamb CR, O'Callaghan MW, Paradis MR. Thoracic radiography in the neonatal foal: a preliminary report. Vet Radiol Ultrasound 1990;31(1):11–6.

11. Sinclair M. Sedation and anesthetic management of foals. In: Sprayberry KA, Robinson NE, editors. Robinson's current therapy in equine medicine, vol. 7. St. Louis (MO): Elsevier; 2015. p. 766–71.

12. Schliewert E-C, Lascola KM, O'Brien RT, et al. Comparison of radiographic and computed tomographic images of the lungs in healthy neonatal foals. Am J Vet Res 2014;76(1):42–52.

13. Lynch KC, Oliveira CR, Matheson JS, et al. Detection of pneumothorax and pleural effusion with horizontal beam radiography. Vet Radiol Ultrasound 2012; 53(1):38–43.

14. Kutasi O, Horvath A, Harnos A, et al. Radiographic assessment of pulmonary fluid clearance in healthy neonatal foals. Vet Radiol Ultrasound 2009;50(6):584–8.

15. Aherne W, Dawkins MJ. The removal of fluid from the pulmonary airways after birth in the rabbit, and the effect on this of prematurity and pre-natal hypoxia. Neonatology 1964;7(4–5):214–29.

16. Bland RD, Hansen TN, Haberkern CM, et al. Lung fluid balance in lambs before and after birth. J Appl Physiol 1982;53(4):992–1004.

17. Barker PM, Olver RE. Invited review: clearance of lung liquid during the perinatal period. J Appl Physiol 2002;93(4):1542–8.

18. Katz C, Bentur L, Elias N. Clinical implication of lung fluid balance in the perinatal period. J Perinatol 2011;31(4):230–5.

19. Christmann U, Livesey LC, Taintor JS, et al. Lung surfactant function and composition in neonatal foals and adult horses. J Vet Intern Med 2006;20(6):1402–7.

20. Koterba AM, Wozniak JA, Kosch PC. Respiratory mechanics of the horse during the first year of life. Respir Physiol 1994;95(1):21–41.

21. Koterba AM, Wozniak JA, Kosch PC. Ventilatory and timing parameters in normal horses at rest up to age one year. Equine Vet J 1995;27(4):257–64.

22. Magnusson L, Spahn DR. New concepts of atelectasis during general anaesthesia. Br J Anaesth 2003;91(1):61–72.

23. Staffieri F, De Monte V, De Marzo C, et al. Effects of two fractions of inspired oxygen on lung aeration and gas exchange in cats under inhalant anaesthesia. Vet Anaesth Analg 2010;37(6):483–90.

24. Wong DM, Alcott CJ, Wang C, et al. Physiologic effects of nasopharyngeal administration of supplemental oxygen at various flow rates in healthy neonatal foals. Am J Vet Res 2010;71(9):1081–8.

25. Rouby JJ, Puybasset L, Nieszkowska A, et al. Acute respiratory distress syndrome: lessons from computed tomography of the whole lung. Crit Care Med 2003;31(4 Suppl):S285–95.

26. Alexander K, Joly H, Blond L, et al. A comparison of computed tomography, computed radiography, and film-screen radiography for the detection of canine pulmonary nodules. Vet Radiol Ultrasound 2012;53(3):258–65.
27. Gattinoni L, Caironi P, Valenza F, et al. The role of CT-scan studies for the diagnosis and therapy of acute respiratory distress syndrome. Clin Chest Med 2006;27(4):559–70.
28. Hill JR, Horner PE, Primack SL. ICU imaging. Clin Chest Med 2008;29(1):59–76.
29. Rubinowitz AN, Siegel MD, Tocino I. Thoracic imaging in the ICU. Crit Care Clin 2007;23(3):539–73.
30. Johnson PJ, LaCarrubba AM, Messer NT, et al. Neonatal respiratory distress and sepsis in the premature foal: challenges with diagnosis and management. Equine Vet Educ 2012;24(9):453–8.
31. Cipone M, Diana A, Gandini G, et al. Use of computed tomography in thoracic diseases of small animals. Vet Res Commun 2003;27:381–4.
32. Prather AB, Berry CR, Thrall DE. Use of radiography in combination with computed tomography for the assessment of noncardiac thoracic disease in the dog and cat. Vet Radiol Ultrasound 2005;46(2):114–21.
33. Lascola KM, O'Brien RT, Wilkins PA, et al. Qualitative and quantitative interpretation of computed tomography of the lungs in healthy neonatal foals. Am J Vet Res 2013;74(9):1239–46.
34. Wion L, Perkins G, Ainsworth DM, et al. Use of computerised tomography to diagnose a Rhodococcus equi mediastinal abscess causing severe respiratory distress in a foal. Equine Vet J 2001;33(5):523–6.
35. Lascola KM, Joslyn SK, O'Brien RT, et al. Comparison of quantitative interpretation of CT images of the lungs in healthy neonatal foals and foals with pulmonary disease – preliminary findings. Proceedings of the 32nd Symposium of the Veterinary Comparative Respiratory Society. Kennett Square (PA), October 25–29, 2014.
36. Wilkins PA, Lascola KM. Update on interstitial pneumonia. Vet Clin North Am Equine Pract 2015;31(1):137–57.
37. Oliveira CR, Mitchell MA, O'brien RT. Thoracic computed tomography in feline patients without use of chemical restraint. Vet Radiol Ultrasound 2011;52(4):368–76.
38. Lascola KM, Clark-Price S, O'Brien RT, et al. The use of manual alveolar recruitment maneuvers to eliminate atelectasis artifacts identified on thoracic computed tomography in healthy neonatal foals. Proceedings of the 5th World Equine Airway Symposium/Veterinary Comparative Respiratory Society. Calgary (AB), July 15–17, 2013.
39. Henao-Guerrero N, Ricco C, Jones JC, et al. Comparison of four ventilatory protocols for computed tomography of the thorax in healthy cats. Am J Vet Res 2012; 73(5):646–53.
40. Duff JP, Rosychuk RJ, Joffe AR. The safety and efficacy of sustained inflations as a lung recruitment maneuver in pediatric intensive care unit patients. Intensive Care Med 2007;33(10):1778–86.
41. Boriosi JP, Cohen RA, Summers E, et al. Lung aeration changes after lung recruitment in children with acute lung injury: a feasibility study. Pediatr Pulmonol 2012; 47(8):771–9.
42. Kinns J, Mallinowski R, McEvoy F, et al. Special software applications. In: Schwarz T, Saunders J, editors. Veterinary computed tomography, vol. 1. Chichester: John Wiley & Sons Ltd; 2011. p. 67–74.
43. Morandi F, Mattoon JS, Lakritz J, et al. Correlation of helical and incremental high-resolution thin-section computed tomographic and histomorphometric quantitative evaluation of an acute inflammatory response of lungs in dogs. Am J Vet Res 2004;65(8):1114–23.

44. Morandi F, Mattoon JS, Lakritz J, et al. Correlation of helical and incremental high-resolution thin-section computed tomographic imaging with histomorphometric quantitative evaluation of lungs in dogs. Am J Vet Res 2003;64(7):935–44.
45. McEVOY FJ, Buelund L, Strathe AB, et al. Quantitative computed tomography evaluation of pulmonary disease. Vet Radiol Ultrasound 2009;50(1):47–51.
46. Reich H, Moens Y, Braun C, et al. Validation study of an interpolation method for calculating whole lung volumes and masses from reduced numbers of CT-images in ponies. Vet J 2014;202(3):603–7.
47. Joslyn S, Lascola K, O'Brien R. Automated CT lung segmentation technique in healthy and diseased foals. Proceedings of the 17th International Veterinary Radiology Association meeting. Perth (Australia), August 16–21, 2015.
48. Nykamp SG. The equine thorax. In: Thrall: textbook of veterinary diagnostic radiology. vol. 6. 2013. p. 632–48.
49. El Shahed AI, Dargaville PA, Ohlsson A, et al. Surfactant for meconium aspiration syndrome in term and late preterm infants. Cochrane Database Syst Rev 2014;(12). CD002054. Available at: http://onlinelibrary.wiley.com/doi/10.1002/14651858.CD002054.pub3/abstract. Accessed August 3, 2015.
50. Vaala WE, Hamir AN, Dubovi EJ, et al. Fatal, congenitally acquired infection with equine arteritis virus in a neonatal thoroughbred. Equine Vet J 1992;24(2):155–8.
51. del Piero F, Wilkins PA, Lopez JW, et al. Equine viral arteritis in newborn foals: clinical, pathological, serological, microbiological and immunohistochemical observations. Equine Vet J 1997;29(3):178–85.
52. Bernard GR, Artigas A, Brigham KL, et al. The American-European Consensus Conference on ARDS. Definitions, mechanisms, relevant outcomes, and clinical trial coordination. Am J Respir Crit Care Med 1994;149(3):818–24.
53. Dunkel B, Dolente B, Boston RC. Acute lung injury/acute respiratory distress syndrome in 15 foals. Equine Vet J 2005;37(5):435–40.
54. Dunkel B. Acute lung injury and acute respiratory distress syndrome in foals. Clin Tech Equine Pract 2006;5(2):127–33.
55. Lakritz J, Wilson WD, Berry CR, et al. Bronchointerstitial pneumonia and respiratory distress in young horses: clinical, clinicopathologic, radiographic, and pathological findings in 23 cases (1984–1989). J Vet Intern Med 1993;7(5):277–88.
56. Byars TD. Fractured ribs in neonatal foals. AAEP Report, News Notes 1997;13.
57. Jean D, Picandet V, Macieira S, et al. Detection of rib trauma in newborn foals in an equine critical care unit: a comparison of ultrasonography, radiography and physical examination. Equine Vet J 2007;39(2):158–63.
58. Borchers A, van Eps A, Zedler S, et al. Thoracic trauma and post operative lung injury in a neonatal foal. Equine Vet Educ 2009;21(4):186–91.
59. Gotway MB, Reddy GP, Webb WR, et al. High-resolution CT of the lung: patterns of disease and differential diagnoses. Radiol Clin North Am 2005;43(3):513–42.
60. Schwarz T, Johnson V. Lungs and bronchi. In: Schwarz T, Saunders J, editors. Veterinary computed tomography, vol. 1. Chichester: John Wiley & Sons Ltd; 2011. p. 261–77.
61. Zompatori M, Ciccarese F, Fasano L. Overview of current lung imaging in acute respiratory distress syndrome. Eur Respir Rev 2014;23(134):519–30.
62. Mazzei MA, Guerrini S, Cioffi SN, et al. Role of computed tomography in the diagnosis of acute lung injury/acute respiratory distress syndrome. Recenti Prog Med 2012;103(11):459–64.
63. Sheard S, Rao P, Devaraj A. Imaging of acute respiratory distress syndrome. Respir Care 2012;57(4):607–12.

Ultrasonographic Examination of the Equine Neonate: Thorax and Abdomen

 CrossMark

Kim A. Sprayberry, DVM

KEYWORDS

- Neonatal diagnostic imaging • Thoracic ultrasound • Abdominal ultrasound

KEY POINTS

- Diagnostic imaging can substantially augment physical examination findings in neonatal foals.
- Used either in combination with radiography or as a stand-alone imaging modality, ultrasound evaluation of the thoracic and abdominal body cavities is often a high-yield diagnostic undertaking.
- Many of the conditions that afflict neonatal foals are highly amenable to sonographic interrogation, including pneumonia and other changes in the lungs associated with sepsis, systemic inflammatory response syndrome , multiple organ dysfunction, and prematurity; colic arising from both medical and surgical causes; and urinary tract disorders.
- Sonographic imaging is not impaired by intracavitary fluid accumulation, and it reveals abnormalities of both soft tissue and bony origin.
- Adding imaging findings to physical examination and laboratory results aids the veterinarian in detection of intracavitary disease early in evaluation, and this translates into an improved level of both patient care and client care.

IMAGING IS AN IMPORTANT COMPONENT OF A COMPREHENSIVE EXAMINATION

Among the most common owner complaints that prompt presentation of neonatal foals to a veterinarian for evaluation and care are lethargy, failure to nurse, colic, respiratory signs, urinary tract abnormalities, and various manifestations of sepsis and the systemic inflammatory response syndrome. Because foals lack the tolerance for pain or the physiologic compensatory reserves that adult horses can draw on, adopting a passive, wait-and-see approach with a compromised neonate is often

Animal Science Department, Cal Poly University San Luis Obispo, 1 Grand Avenue, San Luis Obispo, CA 93407, USA
E-mail address: kspraybe@calpoly.edu

Vet Clin Equine 31 (2015) 515–543
http://dx.doi.org/10.1016/j.cveq.2015.09.004
0749-0739/15/$ – see front matter Published by Elsevier Inc.

an unrewarding strategy and is considered by some to fall below the present standard of care. The practitioner should conduct a comprehensive examination to return the highest yield possible of relevant information. Combining the visual input of diagnostic imaging with physical examination findings and laboratory results adds thoroughness to the evaluation, not only at the time of initial presentation but also during serial monitoring in follow-up examinations.

Of the diagnostic imaging modalities available for use, ultrasonography, radiography, and, increasingly, computed tomography (CT), can provide important and specific input into medical problems of the neonate. Although the preponderance of cases in which CT was used in equine practice has involved orthopedic or intracranial applications,[1] tomography has recently been used to evaluate the lungs in foals[2–5] and holds promise for investigation of intracavitary diseases in this subset of equine patients in the future. At present, though, its availability is limited; it necessitates use of trained personnel and is generally unavailable after hours, and it requires a foal to be heavily sedated or anesthetized. Radiography and ultrasonography yield complementary information and have specific strengths and weak points in their capabilities, but both types of equipment are portable and can be used as point-of-care testing in the stall.

Diagnostic ultrasound equipment is light and easy to set up; the imaging involves no exposure to ionizing radiation, and owners or other stakeholders present find the real-time images of ultrasound especially compelling and illustrative of explanatory points being made by the veterinarian. From a purely imaging standpoint, ultrasound confers certain advantages that are useful in emergent scenarios: it is not necessary to take multiple views to determine the laterality of a lesion; there are no issues with magnification and loss of resolution with varying film-focal point distance; it is not necessary to obtain the images at peak inspiration; some points inaccessible to radiography (eg, the cranial mediastinum, pleural space, and lung fields lying ventral to the diaphragmatic crura) are easily and sensitively examined with ultrasound; and accumulation of fluid in body cavities or in the lung does not add a general opacity or loss of detail to the images but rather increases the acuity of the imaging. Accumulation of fluid in the pleural or peritoneal cavity, for instance, does not necessitate draining of the fluid and then reimaging so that the lung or visceral organs can be better evaluated, but reveals details of tissue form and function through the fluid—whether lung is atelectic or consolidated, or whether a given segment of intestine surrounded by peritoneal fluid is distended but contractile or distended and adynamic, for example—and also reveals clinically relevant characteristics of the fluid itself—whether it occupies one or both hemothoraces, or whether it is acellular and consistent with a transudate or cell-dense and likely to be hemothorax or exudate, to site 2 examples. In short, gaining skill with sonographic imaging can yield an impressive body of information to what which is obtained through physical examination and laboratory testing.

Sonographic imaging does have some shortcomings, and these will be discussed at relevant points in the following sections detailing specific pathologic conditions. Nevertheless, keeping an ultrasound machine in the practice vehicle or plugged in near the examination room is a convenient, safe, and rapid way to add significantly to the body of information derived from the physical examination. At initial evaluation, and later, during serial monitoring as the foal responds to treatment or morbidity progresses, the value of sonographic imaging to the examining veterinarian is hard to overstate and is the focus of this article. The reader is directed to other sources for details of treatment.

REVIEW OF ACOUSTIC-WAVE BEHAVIOR

Acoustic waves are generated by high-frequency vibration of small crystals that have the quality of being piezoelectric. The word piezoelectric is a derivation of the Greek *piezein*, for press or squeeze, and applies here because a piezoelectric material is one in which charge develops across the surface of the crystal if the crystals are deformed (compressed) by the application of mechanical force. This effect is reversible, and the converse is also true: if electrical charge is applied to the crystal, it will deform slightly the surface configuration of the crystal. When electric current passes into a piezoelectric crystal, these surface deformations give rise to vibrations, and the vibrations generate high-frequency sound waves. Succinctly stated, a piezoelectric material takes electrical energy and converts it to wave energy and takes wave energy and converts it back to electrical energy. In ultrasound transducers, piezoelectric crystals (usually quartz) receive electrical current, vibrate at frequencies unique to their thickness and configuration, and direct pulses of the wave energy into the body. The acoustic waves travel longitudinally away from the transducer and penetrate tissues to depths determined by the wave frequency and tissue impedance. Some of the energy is scattered, and some is reflected back toward the transducer. The time it takes for an echoed pulse to arrive back at the transducer after being emitted is translated by the machine into depth. The ultrasound machine's hardware creates images on the basis of these returning wave echoes in the same way that bats' brains process returning echoes into an image of nearby insect prey. High-frequency sounds are emitted by the bat through its mouth or nose and travel through the air in waves, bouncing off any structures they encounter. After emitting the sound, the bat listens to the returning echoes. The bat's brain processes these echo patterns to construct an image in the same way that the brains of other animals create images from visual information. The processing is unconscious, but the bat perceives echoes that take a longer time to return as distance. If returning echoes reach the bat's left ear before its right ear, it perceives the insect to be to the bat's left. The echoes enable the animal to perceive an insect's vertical position, its size, and in which direction it is traveling, plus distinguish prey echoes from those it receives as background clutter. The return patterns of a pulse of acoustic echoes to the piezoelectric crystals likewise sensitively convey information about organs' depth, location, position, and density.[6,7]

Ultrasound waves are not qualitatively different from the sound waves that can be detected by animals and humans, but are simply higher frequencies than can be detected by the ossicles and other sound detection mechanisms in the middle and inner ear. Healthy young adult humans can hear sound frequencies in the range of 20 Hz to 20,000 Hz, or 20 kHz. Most equine diagnostic ultrasound is conducted using frequencies in the range of 2 to 12 MHz (1 MHz = 1 million vibrations/s).

One of the physical properties of acoustic waves is that they are reflected at any interface where the acoustic impedance of 2 neighboring tissues differs significantly. This principle is relevant for areas in the body where a soft tissue (lower impedance) lies next to a tissue containing gas or to a bony structure (high impedance). Because the generating of a sonographic image depends on the acoustic waves entering and passing through a tissue before returning to the transducer, reflection of the waves at the surface of an organ prevents imaging of any part of that structure below the surface. An acoustic beam aimed at the lungs will traverse the chest wall, parietal pleura, and visceral pleura, and then encounter inflated alveoli. At that interface, the beam is bounced back to the transducer and yields no information about tissue deep to the first millimeter of alveolar tissue. The image yielded by this is a series of parallel white lines called reverberation artifact (**Fig. 1**). In foals with pulmonary disease, lesions

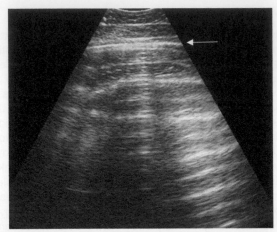

Fig. 1. Sonogram of healthy lung. Near-100% reflection of the acoustic beam at the surface of air-filled alveoli just below the visceral pleura (*arrow*) results in generation of the artifactual white lines, which yield no information about the tissue other than that there is a gas interface at the pleura. This image was obtained with a convex transducer operating at 5 MHz with a display depth of 12 cm.

deep to a layer of aerated alveoli will be obscured from detection for this reason. Lesions that do extend to the periphery of the lung cause no reverberation artifact but instead yield detailed images. Similarly, in the intestinal tract, waves contacting gas at the bowel wall are reflected without providing an image of anything except the wall itself. Areas of subcutaneous emphysema preclude the imaging of any structures deep to the skin by the same concept.

EQUIPMENT USED FOR IMAGING FOALS

Transducers are classified according to the internal arrangement of the crystal elements and according to their frequency. Transducers come in linear, curved, or curvilinear, and phased-array sector configurations. In linear array transducers, the crystals are arranged one next to the other, in a line. These probes create a rectangle-shaped image of high detail but shallow depth. Curved or curvilinear transducers also contain crystals placed next to each other in a linear fashion, but they have a curved footprint; these probes generate a wedge-shaped beam and image. Phased-array scanners contain a small group of crystals emitting a beam that is steered into a sector-shaped slice of tissue in front of the probe. These probes scan an area much wider than the probe's footprint, which is useful when tissues, like the heart, must be imaged through a restricted acoustic window such as the narrow intercostal space (ICS). In general, linear array transducers are used most to image tendons and internal reproductive organs, because the structures of interest are close to the probe surface and the probe shape is appropriate for insertion into a tubular space such as the rectum. Curvilinear transducers are most useful for the types of survey imaging done in neonatal foals and effectively penetrate the thoracic and abdominal body cavities. The phased-array sector scanners have a petite, square footprint that enables rotation of the probe so that 90° views can be obtained from the same acoustic window; these transducers are used in imaging of the heart, referred to as echocardiography.

The frequency of acoustic waves used in veterinary diagnostic ultrasound falls in the range of 2 MHz to 12 MHz. The depth to which acoustic waves travel into the body is inversely proportional to frequency, such that the lowest frequencies travel the farthest, and the higher frequencies penetrate only a few centimeters below the skin surface. There is an inherent tradeoff in selecting a frequency at which to image a body part. The short wavelength of high-frequency sound waves means that there are many returning echoes and a resultant high-detail, high-resolution image, but penetration depth into the body is shallow. The long wavelength of low-frequency waves results in lower-resolution images, but these beams will travel over 30 cm into the body from the skin surface. Multiple-frequency probes are now available, and these emit at a range of frequencies, enabling the examiner to interrogate tissues lying at different depths without having to change probes.

Using sound wave energy to create visual images of organs that are hidden from view inside a body cavity is an amazing but operator-dependent technique, unlike CT, MRI, and radiography, in which the equipment controls the imaging once a button is pushed. The images created by the ultrasound machine are dynamic and change with the examiner's hand position. Scanning structures that are less than perpendicular to the incident beam may introduce changes that look like lesions but are actually positioning artifacts. Acoustic beams that contact tissues at a 90° angle have less scattering and more reflection of energy back to the transducer for processing.

The examiner is well served in investing time to review anatomy with regard to normal locations and spatial relationships among the soft tissue organs occupying the body cavities so that interpreting the images can be done with confidence and accuracy. Diagrams from anatomy texts depicting spatial relationships among organs on both the right and the left sides are helpful in this regard.[8]

PREPARING TO ULTRASOUND

The acoustic beam emitted from the ultrasound transducer will be halted by the air trapped in the hair coat, so the body area to be scanned should first be either clipped with electric clippers or generously wetted with warmed rubbing alcohol. Alcohol displaces the air between and beneath hairs and creates a necessary interface for transfer of an incident beam into the body in the presence of hair. If the hair is clipped, ultrasound coupling gel is applied to the skin. Clipping the hair coat is generally recommended and facilitates higher image resolution, but the author prefers not to clip hair in most instances for examining structures in the body cavities, especially in cold climates, making application of generous volumes of rubbing alcohol necessary at times. Application of water to the hair will not yield the same result and is unhelpful for ultrasound imaging. The alcohol should be applied in a unidirectional fashion, in the direction of hair growth; rubbing against the nap will introduce air and defeats the purpose of applying the alcohol. Before applying it to the foal's skin, the rubbing alcohol should be warmed by preplacing 1 to 2 plastic bottles in a bucket of hot water (not by heating in a microwave oven) for a few minutes. Sloshing cold alcohol onto a foal's skin induces justifiable reaction and struggling and will also chill the foal. Allowing the alcohol to warm before applying it to the foal's thorax or abdomen makes the procedure more pleasant for patient and examiner alike. Clipping of the hair is recommended for ultrasound of superficial structures, such as the umbilicus. After the ultrasound examination, the foal should be gently toweled dry.

SONOGRAPHIC SURVEY OF THE THORACIC CAVITY

Once the hair coat has been wetted, the thorax should be visually inspected for plaques of edema or swelling in the chest wall, especially near the costochondral junctions. In a neonatal foal, this should raise suspicion of a rib fracture, and the area should be gently palpated to check for a pain response from the foal or crepitus from fractured rib ends. Foals in which rib fractures are suspected should not be manipulated or handled in any manner that will compress the ribs or sternum. Attendants working with these foals should assist them to stand by lifting from the foal's stifles and elbows rather than by passing an arm under the chest or belly. Rib fractures are a significant source of morbidity and fatality in some practices[9] and appear to be most common in thoroughbred foals, foals born to a primiparous mare, and foals delivered with human assistance, with or without dystocia.[10–12]

The soft tissue structures inside the thorax are viewed in the spaces between the ribs. In neonates, thoracic contents are sensitively surveyed with a microconvex linear transducer operating at frequencies of 4 MHz to 8 MHz. Linear transducers such as those used for transrectal imaging can also yield good images, although some find these images less intuitive to interpret. The author prefers to use a transducer with a microconvex footprint for surveying the organs inside the thorax and a linear transducer operating at 6 MHz to 10 MHz for imaging the ribs and other superficial structures. When a fracture is found, a higher frequency (8–12 MHz) can be used to view the site with maximal detail. Because of the tradeoff between detail and depth, the overarching principle of sonographic imaging is to use the highest available frequency that will penetrate to the depth necessary for any given tissue.

With the foal lying in lateral recumbence and the thoracic skin surface wetted with alcohol, the examiner begins at the cranial-most section of the chest, the thoracic inlet. This area lies deep to the triceps musculature, and the examination commences with the transducer placed on the lateral aspect of the shoulder and parallel to the long axis of the ribs. The transducer should be held perpendicular to the skin surface. The thymus lying in the cranial mediastinal space can be seen by gently pulling the foal's forelimbs forward and aiming the transducer cranially from the third ICS, from either side. Ribs 1 through 4 form struts around the thoracic inlet and cranial mediastinum and lie deep to the triceps musculature. Rib 5 is usually the first rib that can be seen or palpated just caudal to the lateral head of the triceps when the forelimb is in a neutral position. Beginning with the transducer positioned dorsally in each rib interspace, as the examination proceeds caudally rib by rib, the examiner moves it distally slowly and smoothly, keeping the eyes on the ultrasound monitor. The pleural surface can be evaluated for thickness, and the pleural space is evaluated to ensure there is no fluid. The inner limit of the chest wall is delineated by the linear white echo that slides back and forth in the frame (actually dorsally and ventrally with inhalation and exhalation, respectively) with the foal's respiratory excursions. This movement may be subtle in weak, obtunded foals. The moving white line represents the visceral pleura, and the lung is the tissue lying immediately deep to the line. In healthy lung, the series of multiple parallel white lines representing reverberation artifact is seen just below the moving pleural line, yielding no real information about the pulmonary parenchyma. A lesion lying just deep or axial to a zone of inflated lung will be obscured from view.

Unlike normal lung, diseased pulmonary tissue is highly amenable to sonographic interrogation because it does not yield reverberation artifact. Inflammation, fluid accumulation, consolidation of the air spaces and interstitium, and abscess formation all form a favorable medium for transmission of acoustic waves. Pneumonia is discussed further in a later section.

To image the ribs themselves, the transducer is placed directly on top of the rib and the fingers are used to stabilize it there as the probe is drawn distally along the rib arch. Fractures are recognized by a site of discontinuity in the periosteal and endosteal surfaces, and a surrounding area of hypoechoic fluid will be seen adjacent to the site, representing a hematoma (**Fig. 2**). If the fracture involves ribs 4 to 6, the beating myocardial wall may be seen beating against the shard of fractured bone, giving a visually sobering appreciation for the potential lethality of these injuries.

SONOGRAPHIC SURVEY OF THE ABDOMEN

Beginning in the cranial-most aspect of the abdomen, beginning in ICS space 7 on the left side, the first structure to be encountered, lying in contact with the diaphragm, is the liver. Just caudal to that, in ICS 6 to 12, depending on the volume of the gastric contents, lies a curvilinear arc that represents the greater curvature of the stomach (**Fig. 3**). The liquid contents of the neonatal stomach enables viewing of the luminal contents; by about 7 days of age,[13] gas echoes will fill the stomach, limiting evaluation to the mural structures. Immediate caudal to and in contact with the stomach lies the cranial pole of the spleen, which has a solid, stromal architecture and soft tissue echogenicity. The spleen should be more echogenic than the liver; the difference is easily appreciated where the caudal edge of the left liver lobe lies in contact with the stomach and cranial pole of the spleen, in ICS 8 to 10 on the left side. The spleen can be viewed from ICS 7 back to the paralumbar fossa area, depending on the state of splenic contraction or engorgement at the time of examination. The left kidney is a hypoechoic structure lying axial to the spleen from ICS 15 to the caudal border of the paralumbar fossa and can be recognized by the typical oblong shape and the corticomedullary anatomic pattern with the echogenic cortex, hypoecholc medulla, and hyperechoic renal pelvis. In the groin area ventral to the paralumbar fossa and in the area caudal to the fossa, segments of jejunum can be seen. Large colon segments occupy most of the ventral abdomen in all quadrants and, unlike in older foals and adult horses, will be filled with fluid rather than with a sonoreflective gas layer. The urinary bladder is viewed in the caudoventral aspect of the abdomen.

On the right side of the body, again proceeding in a cranial-to-caudal direction, the first structure seen on the abdominal side of the diaphragm, in ICS 7 to 14, is again the liver. The liver lies in the cranioventral and middle regions of the abdomen in these rib spaces and is also seen in the dorsal abdomen at its caudal-most extent in ICS 14. Bile ducts and hepatic blood vessels can be seen in the liver parenchyma, and the

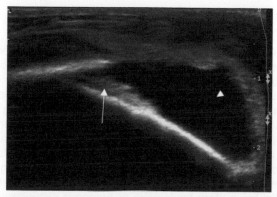

Fig. 2. Sonogram of fractured rib in a neonatal foal. The hematoma formed around the rib ends is organizing, and only anechoic serum (*arrowhead*) is left under the capsule. A patch of fibrin can be seen adherent to the end of the distal fragment (*arrow*). This fracture is characterized by a moderate degree of distraction of the rib ends. Dorsal is to the left. Image obtained with a linear array transducer operating at 6 MHz and with a display depth of 4 cm.

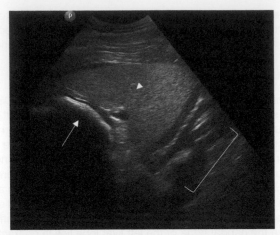

Fig. 3. Sonogram of the cranial part of the left side of the abdomen in a 1-week-old foal. Structures seen are the spleen (*arrowhead*) and the white curvilinear echo of an empty stomach (*arrow*). Also seen in this image are several lengthwise jejunal segments thickened with mural edema (*bracket*). Image obtained with a macroconvex transducer operating at 5 MHz with a display depth of 14 cm.

sharpness of the lobe edges and echogenicity of the parenchyma can be appreciated. Caudal and ventral to the liver in ICS 7 to 12, the examiner will see the long white curvilinear echo corresponding with the right dorsal colon. Beginning in about ICS 10, the duodenum can be viewed in transverse section lying in the dorsal surface of the right dorsal colon and the ventral and caudal margin of the liver. To appreciate the structure, it may be necessary to keep the transducer still and observe for several moments until the duodenum goes through a relaxation-contraction cycle, as duodenal motility is typically intermittent. The duodenum can be seen as far caudally as the cranial margin of the paralumbar fossa, lying ventral to the right kidney and dorsal to the base of the cecum. Moving the transducer ventrally from the right kidney, the examiner can view portions of the cecal body and ventral large colon segments.

DISEASES OF THE THORAX
Pulmonary Abnormalities

Many compromised neonatal foals have pneumonia, whether or not it causes the clinical signs most noticeable to the client. Improper technique for bottle feeding the foal or attempts to nurse by a weak or premature or hypothermic foal can result in aspiration pneumonia. Severe aspiration pneumonitis may be seen in foals that inhaled meconium-contaminated amniotic fluid while gasping during a dystocic birth. Pneumonia is also common in septic foals,[14–16] and in these patients, it should be assumed to be present and treated empirically with a broad-spectrum antimicrobial regimen that has activity against gram-negative bacteria.[17] In hospitalized foals, protracted recumbence can predispose to or exacerbate microbial lung colonization.

The routes of exposure for pneumonia in a newborn foal are well described and include as a partial list in utero bacteremia or fungemia secondary to placentitis in the dam[18]; in utero infection with equine herpesvirus; aspiration of infectious amniotic fluid during gestation in a mare with placentitis; postpartum viral infection; or postpartum bacteremia from pathogen invasion at the portals of the respiratory tract itself, the umbilicus, or the gastrointestinal tract. After a bacteremic event and multisystemic showering, pneumonia may persist as a focal infection and the chief clinical problem. The systemic inflammatory response to microbial infection in the lungs or elsewhere involves some combination of fever, tachypnea/hyperventilation, tachycardia, and changes in immature or mature neutrophil numbers on the hemogram. These adaptive responses are familiar to veterinarians and denote immune recognition of microbial invasion and activation of containment and clearance mechanisms.

In contrast, in some foals, inflammation in the lung itself or at some other site in the body elicits an acute syndrome of devastating, global, self-amplifying, and uncontrolled activation of proinflammatory pathways that manifests predominantly in the lungs. These pathways result in injury of both endothelial and epithelial cells in the lung such that the compartments these cells enclose, the pulmonary capillaries and alveoli, respectively, leak. The lower airspaces and lung interstitium flood with cells, proteinaceous fluid, necrotic material, and fibrin, causing rapidly progressive respiratory distress and hypoxemia, with attendant increases in morbidity and mortality. Acute lung injury (ALI) and acute respiratory distress syndrome (ARDS) are clinical stages in the continuum of severe pulmonary dysfunction that develops with this flooding of fluid and cellular debris into the alveolar spaces and interstitium.[19,20]

Radiographic signs of the pulmonary edema of ALI and ARDS are a generalized opacity and loss of detail along with the appearance of a diffuse alveolar pattern with air bronchograms. Air bronchograms develop when gas-filled airways that have escaped the flooding affecting the alveolar and interstitial spaces stand out against the white, more radiodense areas of infiltration that they course through.[21,22] Radiographic patterns reported in foals with ALI or ARDS include alveolar pattern and mixed alveolar + bronchointerstitial pattern.[23] The sonographic appearance of ALI- or ARDS-associated pulmonary edema on ultrasound is that of a diffuse, unbounded sheet of echogenic infiltration seen especially in the dorsocaudal lung fields.[24] This sonographic infiltrative pattern is highly recognizable but does not permit appreciation of tissue details (**Fig. 4**).

Of the several definition points that must be met in the diagnosis of ALI or ARDS, one involves radiographic detection of infiltrative change in both lungs, and one involves

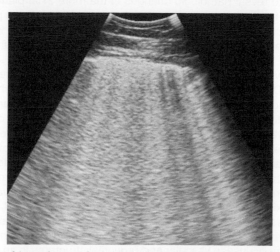

Fig. 4. Sonogram of lung from a foal with NARDS. The lower air spaces and interstitium become flooded with cells and fluid secondary to epithelial and endothelial damage in the wake of severe systemic inflammation. Image obtained with a macroconvex transducer operating at 5 MHz with a display depth of 10 cm.

determination of the $Pao_2:Fio_2$ ratio as an index of the degree of oxygenation impairment. By consensus among a panel of veterinary clinicians and criticalists[25] who met for the purpose of revising for animal use the guidelines established for diagnosing ALI and ARDs in humans,[26] ALI in veterinary patients was defined as a $Pao_2:Fio_2$ ratio less than or equal to 300 and ARDS was defined as a $Pao_2:Fio_2$ ratio less than or equal to 200. To underscore the severity of pulmonary injury necessary to result in these values, it should be appreciated that a healthy adult horse breathing air near sea level has a ratio of approximately 476, as calculated from a Pao_2 of 100 mm Hg and inspired oxygen fraction in atmospheric air of 21%: 100 mm Hg $\div$ 0.21 mm Hg = 476.

The panel further determined that, given the lower range of arterial oxygen tension that prevails for the first week of postnatal life in healthy foals, compared with adult horses, and the fact that arterial blood sampling is performed with foals restrained in lateral recumbency, different reference ranges for Pao_2 and hence for the defining of hypoxemia should be used. The syndromes of ALI and ARDS in neonatal foals were thus given the separate designations of NALI and NARDS.[25] The age-adapted cutoff value for neonatal acute lung injury (NALI) is 175 and for equine neonatal acute respiratory distress syndrome (NARDS) is 115. Ratios in healthy foals are greater than 300.

Although the discussion in this article is weighted toward infectious causes of pneumonia and NARDS, it bears repeating that it is an inflammatory response, not just infection, that triggers the life-threatening escalation in immune response that results in NALI and NARDS. Conditions causing direct injury to pulmonary tissue (eg, traumatic chest injury; pneumonia of bacterial, viral, or fungal origin[27,28]; and aspiration of gastrointestinal contents) as well as diseases that injure the lung indirectly by inciting a massive inflammatory response elsewhere in the body (sepsis, disseminated intravascular coagulation (DIC), traumatic injury to body regions other than the lung, and repeated blood transfusion[23]) have all incited ALI and ARDS.

The lung's responses to infection tend to be similar. These changes will be detected with ultrasound if they extend to the lung surface, but because of the qualitative commonalities in response, sonographic changes do not replace microbial culture and other clinicopathologic testing in the diagnostic workup. In addition, radiography may be needed to reveal pathologic changes in the more axial planes of the chest, which are hidden from sonographic detection by aerated tissue in the periphery. However, sonographic imaging of the chest can reveal pulmonary change well before there are any accompanying clinical signs, giving the veterinarian an earlier intervention window.

In foals that have a typical response to pulmonary infection (ie, one uncomplicated by NALI or NARDS), the earliest evidence of pneumonia may be thickening of the visceral pleura and the appearance of echogenic (white) projections arrayed vertically, or perpendicular to, the surface of the lung (**Fig. 5**). These lesions are called comet-tail lesions and are created by focal thickening, with cells and fluid, in the visceral pleura. In more established cases of pneumonia, the influx of cells and exudative fluid into the infected tissue causes consolidation, meaning that the lower airspaces take on soft tissue density rather than being filled with air. In this typical type of immune response and cell infiltration, neutrophils and other immune cells navigate toward the infection site by chemotaxis and exit the vascular space via the process of diapedesis, but the alveolar walls and pulmonary endothelium remain intact. Because there is no air to generate reverberation artifact at the lung surface, ultrasound can yield a detailed image of the normally unseen vascular and bronchial structures in an area of atelectic or consolidated lung (**Fig. 6**). Although air bronchograms are not sonographically appreciable with pulmonary edema, as they are radiographically, air-filled lower bronchi and bronchioles can be seen with ultrasound in consolidated lung, appearing

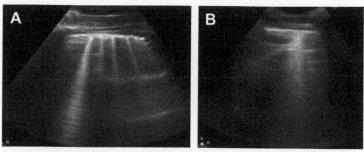

Fig. 5. Sonograms of the left lung of a foal with septicemia and pneumonia. (*A*) Earliest changes noted during serial ultrasound monitoring: pleural thickening and comet-tail lesions extending into the pulmonary parenchyma are seen. (*B*) Same lung 8 hours later. The discrete comet tails have begun broadening and coalescing, indicating progression of infection and pulmonary change. A similar change will also be seen in the dependent lung in foals left in lateral recumbence without frequent turning. Images obtained with a macroconvex tranducer at 5 MHz with a display depth of 14 cm.

as linear or branching hyperechoic structures. The lobar shape and edged borders of the lungs can also be appreciated in lung that is consolidated or atelectic. Containment and organization of infection into an abscess are also sensitively detected sonographically, as long as the abscess borders extend to the pleural surface (**Fig. 7**). Bright white gas echoes seen in areas of consolidated lung may represent the border between consolidated and aerated tissue or may represent islands of aerated alveoli or foci of gas-producing anaerobic bacteria. Pulmonary edema, as develops with left heart failure or from noncardiogenic causes such as NALI or NARDS, appears on ultrasound as a diffuse sheet of homogeneous echogenic material extending to the pleural surface, without boundaries or localizing characteristics (see **Fig. 4**).

A foal being treated and managed for sepsis that has an acute deterioration in clinical status and in which arterial blood gas reveals hypoxemia should be scanned for

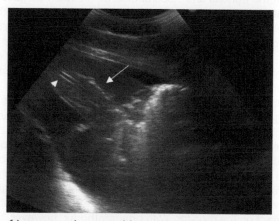

Fig. 6. Sonogram of lung near the ventral lung margin. This lung is atelectatic, which can appear similar to consolidated lung. Easily appreciated are the lung's lobar configuration and details of interior pulmonary parenchyma, made possible by the absence of aerated alveoli. The lung is surrounded by anechoic pleural fluid. An air-filled bronchiole can be seen (*arrow*) along with the parallel walls of a pulmonary blood vessel (*arrowhead*). Dorsal is to the right of this image.

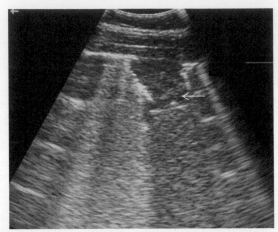

Fig. 7. Sonogram of lung in a foal with pneumonia that is progressing in severity. This view of lung tissue contains areas of normally aerated parenchyma (where there is reverberation artifact), areas of infiltration with cells or edema (diffuse to broad comet tails), and an irregularly shaped focus of developing pulmonary abscess or consolidation (*arrow*). This lesion is appreciable because it extends to the visceral pleura.

lung changes, and appearance of this diffuse pattern of interstitial infiltration that denotes interstitial edema should prompt revisiting of the treatment regimen to include measures aimed at contravening the development of NALI. Detection of these sonographic changes is a good indication for additional imaging with radiography to provide additional information about the distribution and severity of interstitial flooding.

Pleural Space Abnormalities

The pleural space merits evaluation as its own compartment inside the thorax. Because in health the parietal and visceral pleurae maintain contact with each other during both the inflation and the deflation phases of lung movement, the pleural space is really only a potential space where the pressure is maintained at a subatmospheric level, and it should be empty save for a small volume of anechoic fluid that may or may not be detected sonographically. When seen, this small volume of fluid is often detected ventrally and caudal to the heart.[29] Imaging of the chest should reveal the glide sign in all areas, confirming that the dorsal part of the pleural space is devoid of gas and the ventral part is devoid of free fluid. This movement is called the glide sign. The glide sign will not be evident in the ventral aspect of the pleural cavity if there is accumulation of fluid and will be missing from the dorsal aspect of the pleural cavity if there is free gas, or pneumothorax. The presence of effusion or blood in the pleural cavity is easy to detect. With practice and repetition, free gas in the dorsal part of the pleural cavity can also be confirmed sonographically. The ultrasound probe should be placed in the dorsal-most extent of an ICS and held motionless while the lung excursions are observed; as it does inside alveoli, gas free in the pleural cavity will yield reverberation artifact on the monitor. With pneumothorax, however, the parallel white lines of artifact do not move back and forth with the lung, but rather are stationary. Moving the probe ventrally in the same ICS very slowly should reveal a point at which the gliding lung surface enters the ventral side of the frame. That point denotes the extent of the cap of free air in the pleural space. Pneumothorax does not always necessitate intervention; diagnosis of the site of escaping air and very close monitoring of the foal are obviously indicated, but clinical signs, anxiety level (the foal's), and blood gas values should be used to determine at what point or whether the air should be removed.

Rib fractures often lacerate small or large intercostal blood vessels along with the parietal pleura and can cause mild or life-threatening hemothorax. The clinical signs associated with internal hemorrhage may actually be the first indication of broken ribs. Active bleeding in either body cavity has a signature sonographic appearance, deemed the smoke sign (**Fig. 8**). The term refers to the flow pattern of blood exiting an artery or vein: the examiner can usually appreciate constant movement, with the echogenic free fluid swirling into circles and curliques around the lungs and heart. Once a thrombus has formed at the site of bleeding, stationary blood inside a body cavity quickly compartmentalizes, with the heavy, heme-laden erythrocytes settling and being reabsorbed for recycling by the body, and the anechoic serum remaining evident. Scanning at this point reveals only an accumulation of anechoic fluid. It should be mentioned that any fluids with a high cell content have a similar appearance on ultrasound: it is not always possible to differentiate blood from exudate. However, exudate inside a body has no mechanism for self-propagated movement, and the swirling, dynamic appearance of a moving cell-dense fluid inside the chest is strongly suggestive of, if not pathognomonic for, hemothorax.

Laceration of the diaphragm and bowel herniation is another complication of rib fractures. In the author's experience, hemothorax, hemoabdomen, or both should arouse suspicion of diaphragmatic laceration or rupture, and the cavitary hemorrhage may be appreciated as the sole finding, before abdominal organs actually move into the pleural cavity (**Fig. 9**). Therefore, foals with hemothorax should be scanned carefully for rib fractures at initial evaluation, and the finding also warrants reexamination at least daily for several days afterward to ensure no such additional complications have arisen. The ends of the fractured ribs can be very sharp, and the lung surface is lacerated on these bony projections while sliding dorsally and ventrally during ventilation, leading to bleeding in the lung parenchyma, or pulmonary contusion (**Figs. 10** and **11**). The most dangerous complication of rib fractures arises when the involved ribs are ribs 4 through 7, those lying adjacent to the heart. Because of the arch of the proximal segments of the ribs, a complete fracture near the costochondral junction results

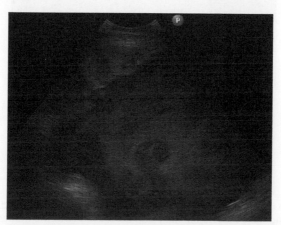

Fig. 8. Sonogram of hemorrhage in a foal with rib fractures and diaphragmatic laceration. Notice the swirl and curlique pattern in the echogenic, cell-dense fluid. Movement of the blood giving rise to the swirling in real time is called the smoke sign.

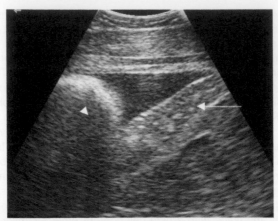

Fig. 9. Sonogram from a foal with a diaphragmatic laceration from rib fractures and herniation of large intestine into the pleural space. The curved white echo (*arrowhead*) is that of a viscus lying between the diaphragm (*arrow*) and chest wall. In this view, the lung is displaced to the left and out of view by the viscus. The liver is to the right of the diaphragm, and the pleural cavity is to the left.

in the distal fragment displacing axially, where its tip becomes an instrument of potentially lethal cardiac injury. Cardiac contusion or laceration is usually a fatal and terminal event; sonographic viewing of the heart beating against a sharp bone shard should prompt discussion of surgery with the owners about the option of immobilizing the fractures that put the foal at risk for cardiac puncture. Treatment recommendations for conservative management of fractured ribs involve enforced exercise restriction for varying lengths of time, often 14 to 21 days. Ultrasound is useful in following the organization and maturation of the hematomas that develop over the fractured rib

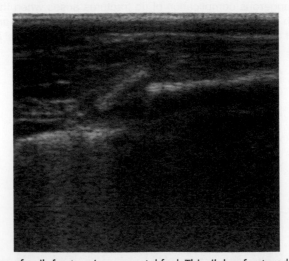

Fig. 10. Sonogram of a rib fracture in a neonatal foal. This rib has fractured at 2 sites, leaving a small floating fragment that is minimally displaced. Even with the modest degree of bony displacement, the comet-tail lesions below the site denote focal hemorrhage in the underlying lung. Dorsal is to the left. Image obtained with a linear array transducer operating at 6 MHz with a display depth of 6 cm.

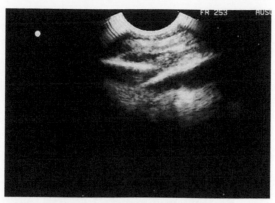

Fig. 11. Sonogram of a fractured rib end piercing and lacerating underlying lung. The heart is protected from similar injury by the lung everywhere but in ribs 3 through 7, where the cardiac notch in the lung lobes leaves the myocardium beating against the parietal pleura and underlying ribs. A fractured rib with this configuration and angle of displacement lying next to the heart would carry a significant risk of fatality.

ends, an important structure in the healing process that cannot be seen in useful detail radiographically; when the hematomas are well-organized and stable, they create a smooth rounded knob that lies between the bone and any neighboring soft tissues, protecting the latter (**Fig. 12**). Formation of a fibrous union between the bone ends can also be verified and followed sonographically (**Fig. 13**).

The Cranial Mediastinum

The mediastinum is the midline space in the thorax lying between the 2 pleural cavities and created by the medial portions of the left and right parietal pleurae coming into proximity. In the midline space created by these structures lie multiple unpaired structures, including the esophagus, lower trachea, heart, thymus, caudal vena cava, azygous vein, and lymph nodes, among a few other structures. Ultrasonography of the heart, or echocardiography, is a complex undertaking that merits its own treatment and is outside the focus of this article, but basic 4-chamber views of the heart can easily be imaged in the window provided by the cardiac notch, in ICS 3 to 5, in the right lung.

The most common reason for viewing structures in the cranial mediastinal space is to investigate whether there is fluid in the pleural space. In horses with pleuropneumonia, the cranial mediastinum is a site where exudate and infective material can organize into an abscess. In foals and in animals up to about 2 years of age, the thymus can be seen in this site. It is useful to practice imaging this space in both recumbent and standing animals. For a compromised neonatal foal, the cranial mediastinal space can be viewed by lying the foal in left lateral recumbence and gently pulling the right (upper) forelimb forward. The transducer is placed in the right third ICS and aimed toward the opposite elbow and cranially. Effusion in that location will appear as an accumulation of anechoic fluid, while the thymus is a loosely organized hypoechoic soft tissue structure.

DISEASES OF THE ABDOMEN
Gastrointestinal Tract Disease

The gastrointestinal tract is susceptible to injury resulting from any of the major morbid conditions affecting more seriously compromised newborn foals: prematurity,

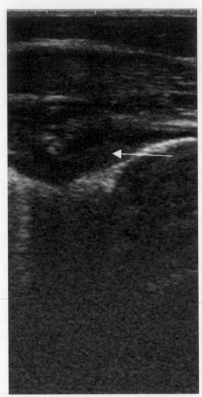

Fig. 12. Sonogram of the distracted ends of a fractured rib with a surrounding hematoma in a neonatal foal. The underlying lung is lacerated but is protected from further injury by the moving rib ends by the thick wall of the organizing hematoma (*arrow*). Dorsal is to the left. Image obtained with a linear array transducer operating at 5 MHz with a display depth of 6 cm.

asphyxia-related injury, and septicemia can all induce injury and dysfunction, including diarrhea, in the gastrointestinal tract.[30,31] All can lead to functional failure of the blood-mucosal barrier as well as to motility failure, and these 2 problems are responsible for many of the clinical signs and abnormalities affecting the seriously compromised neonate. The gastrointestinal tract constitutes both a significant potential portal of entry for microbes and a vulnerable target for bacteremic showering by pathogens that entered the body by another route.[31] It is common to find sonographic abnormalities in the abdomen of compromised foals, with or without colic.

The author approaches sonographic survey of the foal abdomen by imaging all the structures mentioned in the Abdominal Survey section while making sure to record several primary aspects of visceral anatomy and function: the mural width of the small and large intestine walls; the sonographic character of the mural layers, whatever their measured thickness; the nature of the luminal contents; and the contractility patterns, in any discrete segment of interest and in the context of overall tract motility. Particularly with gastrointestinal problems, which can be fulminant and rapidly changing, imaging is most helpful when the foal can be scanned serially over a certain time interval so that change can be detected. Also, the visual observations must be interpreted in light of concurrent changes in physical status, laboratory test values, and response to treatment. That said, foals with colic or other signs referable to the abdomen often do

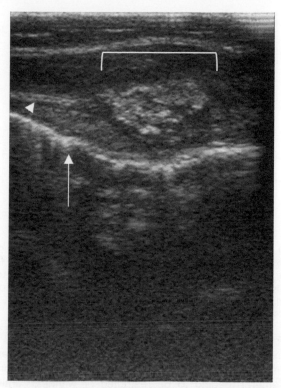

Fig. 13. Sonogram from a foal with several fractured ribs. Shown is the right sixth rib at the fracture site. The hematoma is resorbing, and the fracture ends have formed an early fibrous union (*bracket*). The proximal fragment enters the image from the left (*arrowhead*). The underlying lung still has evidence of contusion injury, with a thickened visceral pleura (*arrow*) and underlying pattern consistent with extravasated blood. Dorsal is to the left. Image obtained with a linear array transducer operating at 5 MHz and with a display depth of 6 cm.

have abnormalities involving the gastrointestinal tract and other abdominal viscera on ultrasound. Surgical and medical lesions in the intestinal tract can manifest very similarly.

The most common indicator of gastrointestinal tract injury from sepsis or hypoxic-ischemic insult in a newborn foal is motility failure. Gastroduodenal ileus results in a distended, hypomotile stomach and duodenum filled with milk or residual fluid that is not proceeding down the tract (**Fig. 14**). When the stomach is distended and atonic, the duodenum will usually be found in a similar state. Normal small intestinal mural thickness in foals is less than or equal to 3 mm,[13,32,33] but any time mural width is scrutinized, the qualitative appearance of the viscus wall should also be noted, even if the mural width is normal. Scanning a bowel segment with a higher-frequency probe is needed to distinguish the layers of the bowel wall, but if available, this should be performed to confirm the following normal echo patterns: hyperechoic mucosal surface–hypoechoic mucosa–hyperechoic submucosa–hypoechoic muscularis propria–hyperechoic serosa.[29,32] Appearance of hypoechoic edema in the bowel wall even before there is thickening of the overall dimensions may be seen with strangulating lesions, and the appearance of hyperechoic gas echoes within the wall layers is diagnostic for pneumatosis intestinalis and necrotizing enterocolitis.[34]

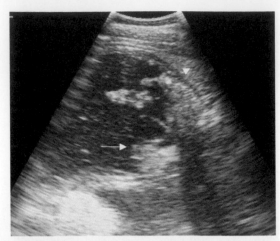

Fig. 14. Sonogram from a neonatal foal with enterocolitis and delayed gastric emptying. An interface between curdled milk (*arrow*) and gas-flecked hypoechoic fluid can be seen causing moderate gastric distension. The spleen (*arrowhead*) is to the right of the stomach in this image. Image obtained with a macroconvex transducer operating at 5 MHz with a display depth of 14 cm.

Detection of distension and delayed emptying of the stomach and duodenum help the veterinarian make several management decisions. First, the distension and atony necessitate placement of an indwelling feeding tube to facilitate decompression every few hours, and enteral feeding to be restricted or withheld, until contractility is restored. Persistent gastric engorgement and absence of propulsive contractions would also prompt addition of partial or total parenteral nutrition, prokinetic agents, gastroprotectants, and antiulcer medications to the regimen, in addition to the antimicrobials, intravenous fluids, and other interventions the foal was receiving. Incorporating imaging as part of morning and evening physical examinations can visually confirm the return of contractility, and the foal's management is modified accordingly.

Gastritis and ulcer formation in neonatal foals are a multifactorial and complex clinical entity, discussion of which is outside the scope of this article, but visceral hypoperfusion secondary to sepsis-associated hypotension or from failure to keep up with the foal's fluid needs, to name 2 examples, likely constitute risk factors for this complication that are unrelated to acidity alone, as ulcers can develop and progress to the point of gastric perforation even while foals are receiving proton pump inhibitors. Reflux of duodenal fluids into the stomach may also injure the mucosa by contact with bile acids. Ulcer formation proceeding to gastric perforation can be clinically silent, especially in recumbent, obtunded foals. Gastric endoscopy is the only definitive method for diagnosing gastric ulcers, but sonographic imaging of the area in the left cranial abdomen where the liver, stomach, and spleen lie in contact can reveal gastric wall edema and serositis as local effects of severe ulcerative gastritis and incipient perforation (**Fig. 15**).

Bacterial and viral pathogens can cause enteritis or enterocolitis in foals beginning on the first day of postnatal life. The sonographic hallmark of enteritis of any cause is the combination of distension, hypomotility (although hypermotility may be seen in the prodromal stages), intestinal walls of normal or thickened width, and hypoechoic-to-echogenic gassy luminal contents (**Fig. 16**). With severe enteritis, transudative-to-exudative fluid may also accumulate in the peritoneal fluid and can set the foal

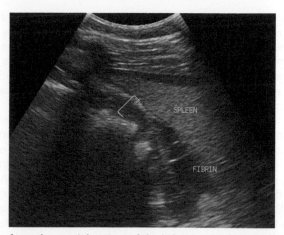

Fig. 15. Sonogram from the cranial region of the left side of a foal's abdomen, in rib spaces 9 and 10. This view features the area where the stomach and spleen lie in proximity and reveals local peritonitis with fine fibrinous adhesions forming between the stomach and spleen. The gastric wall (*bracket*) is thickened with edema and serositis from an ulcer in the process of perforating. This image was obtained with a macroconvex transducer operating at 5 MHz with a display depth of 14 cm.

up for fibrous adhesions in the weeks to months following clinical resolution of the enteritis. The distended small intestine segments are easy to find and form the dominant feature in the affected foal's abdomen. In the prodromal phase of infection, hypermotility rather than hypomotility may be appreciated. The intestinal walls are often of normal width, but may also have an inflamed appearance and be thicker than normal. Enteritis and enterocolitis in newborn foals are severe systemic diseases, attended by dehydration, pain, and marked acid-base and metabolic alterations. The most common causes in newborn foals include bacterial infection (*Clostridium*

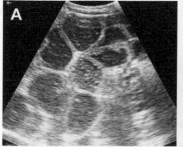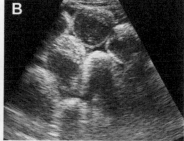

Fig. 16. Sonograms from neonatal foals with small intestinal disease. (*A*) Jejunal segments in a 2-day-old foal with enterocolitis caused by *C perfringens* type A. Although views of jejunum are not always easily seen in healthy neonates, small intestine distension displaces other viscera and makes the affected segments easy to detect. (*B*) Jejunal segments from a 1-week-old foal with small intestine volvulus. In this foal, the intestine walls have not become severely thickened from venous congestion, but the effects of profound ileus can be appreciated in the settling out of the solids in the luminal contents. The top portion of the image represents the abdominal floor. Both images were obtained with a convex transducer operating at 5 MHz with a display depth of 15 cm.

perfringens, Clostridium difficile, Enterococcus durans, and *Salmonella* spp) and viral infection (rotavirus, coronavirus). Less common microbial pathogens that have been reported in diarrheic foals include *Aeromonas hydrophila, Bacteroides fragilis, Cryptosporidium parvum,* and adenovirus.[30] Blood work in foals with enteritis usually features leukopenia with neutropenia, a feature of the mucosal barrier compromise, and fever is often also found, although fever in neonatal foals is not a reliable clinical finding, and its absence should not be relied on to rule out serious illness.

The sonographic appearance of strangulated small intestine is similar to that of enteritis or enterocolitis,[35] but venous congestion in the strangulated bowel wall will lead to a progressive increase in mural width and engorgement of mesenteric vasculature over time (see **Fig. 16**). Causes of intestinal strangulation in neonatal foals include volvulus; incarceration through a mesenteric rent or by a congenital anomaly such as Meckel diverticulum; and herniation through the inguinal ring or a rupture in the diaphragm. Because the initial appearance of strangulated small intestine may closely resemble that of enteritis, it is necessary to incorporate additional information into the evaluation in determining whether the foal requires surgical intervention. Analysis of peritoneal fluid, blood work, physical status, and response to analgesics is necessary for making this determination.

Intestinal intussusception has been well described as a cause of colic in foals, but this disorder is more common in foals several months of age and older than in neonatal foals. Development of intussusception arises from differences in motility between neighboring segments of bowel and may be associated with many causes, including enteritis, administration of the prokinetic neostigmine, and parasitism. Intussuscepted intestine has a typical and easily recognizable sonographic appearance formed from the concentric layering of one bowel segment (the intussusceptum) inside an outer segment (the intussuscipiens; **Fig. 17**).[36,37] Intussusceptions can be jejunojejunal, ileal-ileal, ileocecal, cecocolic, or cecocecal.[37] Clinical signs and severity of colic resulting from intussusception depend on length of involved bowel segment and whether the mesenteric blood vessels attached to the intussusceptum are obstructed. It is generally accepted that diagnosis of an intussusception automatically warrants surgical correction, and in older foals and horses, this is likely true. However, a recent report[33] detailing the existence of intussusceptions as an incidental finding in healthy, asymptomatic standardbred foals confirms that in neonates this is not always true. The findings in that study corroborate observations by the author, who has observed

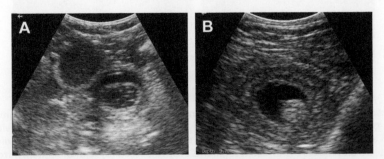

Fig. 17. Sonograms of 2 types of intussusception. (*A*) Jejunojejunal intussusception in a hospitalized neonate. This image was obtained in the caudal abdomen of the foal while it was positioned in right lateral recumbence. (*B*) Cecocecal intussusception, with the tip of the cecum inverted into the cecal body. This image was obtained in a yearling colt but is included here for example. Image obtained near ventral midline with horse standing.

jejunojejunal intussusceptions arising in multiples in hospitalized foals and resolving spontaneously (unpublished data, 2012).

Most causes of colic in neonatal foals are medical problems of the gastrointestinal tract. In a recent retrospective study[35] of colic in 137 neonatal foals (defined as <30 days of age; median age, 2 days) at a university referral hospital, 89% of the foals had conditions that were managed medically. For all 137 foals, enterocolitis, meconium-related colic, and transient colic for which a cause was not determined but which was managed medically were the 3 most common diagnoses. In the 11% of foals that underwent surgery for colic, small intestine strangulating obstruction was the most frequent diagnosis, with volvulus, intussusception, and mesenteric rent comprising most of these cases.

Meconium, a sterile concretion of intestinal cells and secretions, accumulates in the intestine during gestation and becomes sufficiently tenacious or inspissated in some foals that it becomes impacted in the large intestine or rectum and causes obstruction. In meconium impaction or retention, ultrasound is sensitive at detecting the impacted colon segment and the length or extent of the retained luminal material (**Fig. 18**). Change in the appearance of the mass can be monitored sonographically after administration of enteral fluids or an enema. The affected colon segments and retained pellets or logs are usually detected in the caudal part of the abdomen. In the 2013 retrospective mentioned previously,[35] ultrasound was helpful in distinguishing large intestinal from small intestinal disease, and, within a portion of the intestine, types of disease. Distended, hypodynamic small intestine was seen more frequently with strangulating lesions, enterocolitis, and necrotizing enterocolitis than in those with meconium-associated colic. Within the large intestine, fluid distension was seen more frequently in foals with enterocolitis and necrotizing enterocolitis than in those with meconium problems. Thickening of the bowel wall was also sensitively detected: mural thickening in the small intestine was seen with strangulating obstructions, enterocolitis, and necrotizing enterolitis, but not with meconium-associated, transient medical colic, or forms of colic deemed "other". Thickening of the large intestine wall was seen only in foals with necrotizing enterocolitis. The fact that mural thickening was seen in foals with strangulating small intestinal lesions and those with inflammatory bowel lesions underscores how sonography is useful at detecting the site of abnormality but must be supported with physical examination and clinicopathologic data in the process of making a definitive diagnosis in these types of diseases. In the scenario of a colicky neonatal foal with thickened small intestine walls, for example, fever, a low white cell count, abnormal serum electrolyte values, and fluid accumulating in both the small and the large intestine would point toward enterocolitis. Severity of pain and response to pain controlling medications are also clinically useful. In this study,[35] neonates with a strangulating small intestine lesion (usually a volvulus) were significantly more likely to have severe pain and continuous pain than foals with medical causes of colic, and fewer foals with strangulating lesions responded to analgesics, compared with those that had medical colic.

Recently, a protocol of focused abdominal scanning designed for use in emergent settings was assessed in horses with colic.[38] In this protocol, abdominal imaging is limited to assessing visceral structures and free peritoneal fluid volume at 7 topographic locations. The technique is deemed FLASH (fast localized abdominal sonography in horses) and has conceptual precedent in human[39] and small animal[40] emergency medicine. The 7 designated imaging windows were selected on the basis of earlier reports of frequent locations for detection of sonographic abnormalities in horses with colic. In this 2011 report of horses with colic,[38] use of the focused technique was quickly learned by individuals who did not have extensive ultrasound

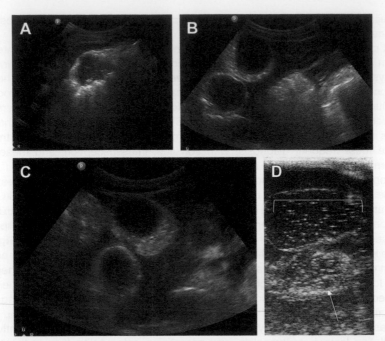

Fig. 18. Sonograms of large intestine in a neonatal foal with meconium-associated colic. (*A*) Longitudinal view of the bowel segment obstructed by the meconium, which is the hypoechoic material with the oblong shape surrounded by intestinal wall that is contracted around the material. Meconium is sonographically hypoechoic to anechoic, despite its solid consistency. (*B*) Same area as in (*A*). The thin layer of echogenic material surrounding the anechoic meconium balls is luminal fluid beginning to accumulate after enteral administration of water and mineral oil and administration of a retention enema. (*C*) The impacted accumulations of meconium are smaller, and the volume of fluid surrounding them in the colonic lumen has increased in the hour since the image in (*B*) was taken. This indicates response to treatment and the process of resolution of the meconium retention. (*D*) The meconium (*bracket*) in this image has a more speckled, echogenic appearance on ultrasound. This image was obtained with a linear array transducer in a foal with hemoabdomen resulting from rib fractures and diaphragm laceration. A thrombus is represented by the echogenic clot lying against the deep surface of this meconium ball (*arrow*).

experience and enabled quick (mean examination time, 10.7 minutes) evaluation and acceptable sensitivity, specificity, and predictive values in horses whose clinical condition made performing a complete abdominal survey impossible. Use of this focused protocol in neonatal foals has not been reported, but will likely be investigated in these patients in the future.

Urinary Tract Abnormalities

Considerable overlap can exist among the clinical signs of gastrointestinal and urinary tract disease. Colic and diarrhea can be seen in diseases of both systems, and ultrasound can help distinguish between gastrointestinal and urinary tract disease. Transitioning of the urogenital system from fetal to postnatal life at the time of birth involves abrupt changes in the umbilical remnant structures, as blood flow ceases entering and exiting the body through the umbilical cord and the roles of urine formation and handling are transferred from the placenta to the foal's organs. The umbilical cord should rupture cleanly a short distance from the foal's abdominal wall, leaving a 1″ to 2″ stump,[41] at which time the vascular structures inside the cord immediately contract and begin occluding further blood flow. Inside the umbilical cord are 4 clinically important structures that can be assessed sonographically: 2 umbilical arteries, 1 umbilical vein, and the urachus. In gestation, these structures are anatomically independent, but are bundled into a cord by an outer adventitial covering.

In thoroughbred foals, the maximum normal cord length has been determined to be less than 84 cm (range, 36–83 cm; mean, 55 cm), with up to 4 twists along its length.[42] Cord length is of clinical relevance because an abnormally long cord can become excessively torsed or wrapped around the fetus' trunk or limbs in utero, strangulating or impinging the structures within it. Upstream dilatation and pressure in the urachus and bladder created by cord impingement can predispose to higher-than-normal intravesicular volume, and bladder rupture, during parturition. A short umbilical cord increases traction on the placenta during parturition and may result in premature placental separation and death for the foal if a human attendant is not present. Short cord length can also create tension on the foal's umbilical area and urachus during and after transit through the birth canal, increasing the risk for tearing and urine leakage postpartum. A subjective appreciation for excessive umbilical cord length can be obtained during sonographic monitoring of the gestating mare. Umbilical cord abnormalities in utero thus can have an important influence on events involving the urogenital system in the neonate.

In the fetal vasculature, the umbilical arteries arise as branches of the pudendal arteries, which are branches of the internal iliac arteries. From their origins on the pudendal arteries in the dorsocaudal aspect of the abdomen, the umbilical arteries flow cranially and ventrally toward the bladder, where each travels on its respective side along the lateral aspect of the bladder. From its entry site at the umbilical stalk, the umbilical vein courses cranially along abdominal midline and into the liver. In the weeks following birth, the umbilical vein atrophies and becomes the cordlike round ligament of the liver, running through the fatty connective tissue of the falciform ligament. The umbilical arteries also undergo involution and atrophic change and become the round ligaments of the bladder. Unlike these vascular remnants, the urachus is not a walled tubular structure, but is merely the potential space running between and around the umbilical blood vessels. In the fetus, the urachus is the conduit for urine flow from fetal bladder to the allantoic cavity. At the time of birth, it should involute and close, and the foal should begin voiding urine through the urethra.

Even though the remnant umbilical arteries course caudally and dorsally toward the bladder, because the bladder lies so close to the ventral abdominal wall in neonates, these structures are still quite superficial with regard to imaging depth. High-resolution images are needed for determining the dimensions of small structures such as arteries and vein, and this is one study in which the author routinely clips the hair. Clipping should include the area around the base of the umbilicus, between the base and the groin, and between the base and the liver. Foals can be scanned standing, in lateral recumbence, or in a semi-dorsal recumbent position. Imaging frequencies in the range of 6 MHz to 10 MHz will yield useful images for this study.

The umbilical arteries and vein should be imaged along their full length. The umbilical vein is observed in the transverse plane and longitudinal plane running from its origin at the umbilical base cranially toward the liver. It should be less than 1 cm in diameter throughout its length, with some narrowing about halfway between the base and the point where the vein merges into the hepatic tissue.[32,43] The arteries are observed by placing the probe at the umbilical base on its caudal surface. At this juncture, the arteries and urachus are seen together in an oblong grouping, and the long-axis diameter there should be less than 2.5 cm. Moving the probe caudally along midline, the urachus will disappear, and the arteries will diverge laterally along the bladder walls. When imaged separately, each umbilical artery remnant in transverse section should be less than 1 cm. It is easier to discern the arteries when the bladder is partially full. Of the structures comprising the umbilical remnant, the urachus is the most commonly infected.[44] Infection appears as soft tissue or echogenic material in the urachal lumen or occupying the tissue spaces around the arteries or urachus. Well-established umbilical infections come to notice by gross thickening, edema, or cellulitis surrounding the umbilical base. Exudate may be dripping from the stalk, or infection may have caused the urachus to become patent again and drip urine. Infection that tracks internally can cause cellulitis of the subcutaneous tissues surrounding the stalk and peritonitis. Internal structures can be infected and have significant sonographic abnormalities even if the external portion of the stalk appears normal.

Sonographic imaging is of great benefit in detecting sites of rupture in the urinary tract and infection of the internal umbilical remnants, the most common causes of urinary tract disease affecting neonates. Leaking of urine into the peritoneal cavity can result from rupture of the ureters, bladder, urethra, or urachus. Underlying conditions that can cause leak are parturition-associated trauma, congenital anomalies, postpartum traumatic injury, strenuous exercise, focal necrosis of the bladder wall, and urachal infection.[45,46]

Foals with uroperitoneum present with one or more of the following well-documented clinical signs: colic, tenesmus secondary to constipation, tachycardia, altered mucous membrane appearance, dehydration, diarrhea, failure to nurse, lethargy, abdominal distension, frequent urinary posturing, and stranguria. Affected foals may also have rapid, shallow breathing secondary to hampering of diaphragmatic contraction by the volume of fluid in the abdomen.[47] Foals usually continue to pass some urine through the urethra as well as through the bladder rent into the abdomen, and it often takes several days after birth for the abdominal distension to become marked enough to prompt veterinary evaluation. When the rupture is in a ureter, the uroperitoneum develops more slowly and takes longer to manifest clinically. The hallmark sonographic appearance of uroperitoneum is voluminous anechoic to hypoechoic fluid in which viscera and mesentery are floating. Some foals with uroperitoneum also develop pleural effusion.[48] If the uroperitoneum is chronic or is associated with rupture of an infected or necrotic urachus, the peritoneal fluid will become more cellular in appearance with the influx of leukocytes. It is not always possible to make out the tear site in the bladder wall, but it can be appreciated in some instances.

The gender predilection toward male foals traditionally reported[49] was not found in 2 more recent retrospective studies on uroperitoneum in foals.[50,51] Moreover, the clinical presentation and serum biochemical abnormalities associated with uroperitoneum may be different in foals hospitalized for sepsis or hypoxic-ischemic injury, in which uroperitoneum arises as one of multiple systemic abnormalities, than they are in foals referred to a hospital with uroperitoneum as the primary complaint.[50] In hospitalized foals, clinical signs can be masked by a neurologically depressed state, and administration of intravenous fluids prevents or blunts the hyponatremia, hypochloremia, and hyperkalemia that have traditionally been strongly associated with uroperitoneum.[49,52] Administration of fluids does not impact the development of high serum creatinine concentration or the usefulness of determining the peritoneal fluid:serum creatinine ratio, with a ratio 2 or greater being diagnostic for uroperitoneum. It is likely that more prevalent use of diagnostic ultrasound has resulted in diagnosis and intervention before the full gamut of biochemical changes can develop. The bladder is the most common site of rupture in the tract, followed by the urachus. In the 2005 retrospective study[51] cited in these paragraphs, the rent in the bladder wall was ventral at about the same frequency as it was dorsal.

Sepsis and focal infections, in the urogenital tract[53] and elsewhere in the body, are important risk factors for uroperitoneum, irrespective of whether a foal is hospitalized.[50,51] In these foals, rupture of the bladder or urachal remnant is related to infection or necrosis rather than to traumatic rupture during parturition. It is not uncommon to detect uroperitoneum in a septic or bedridden foal one or more days into hospitalization when it was not present at admission. It is advisable to place and properly maintain an indwelling urinary catheter in nonambulatory foals to prevent urine stasis and pressure in the bladder, and broad-spectrum antimicrobial coverage would be an expected part of the treatment regimen of any foal in this state. Daily to twice-daily sonographic imaging of the abdomen during the course of hospitalization enables detection of even a modest volume of free peritoneal fluid, days before abdominal distension, colic, or some of the other clinical signs become evident. The bladder is the most common site of rupture in the tract, followed by the urachus. In the 2005 retrospective study[51] cited in these paragraphs, the rent in the bladder wall was ventral at about the same frequency as it was dorsal. Excellent practical guides on scanning technique for the umbilical remnants are available.[54]

The term navel ill has traditionally been used in reference to septic polyarthritis thought to result from pathogens' gaining entrance to the body through the umbilicus. Although the umbilicus can indeed serve as an access point for pathogens, it is now recognized that the gastrointestinal tract and other portals are often the chief entry point, and the umbilical structures can become infected by bacteremic showering along with other tissues. The most common reported bacterial isolates from omphalitis or omphalophlebitis specimens are Escherichia coli and Streptococcus zooepidemicus.[44,55,56] Infection with C perfringens has also been reported, as a result of either direct invasion from the environment or bacterial translocation from the intestinal tract.[55] A 2007 report[57] revealed Clostridium sordelli as a cause of fulminant omphalitis, peritonitis, and death in 8 foals.

Bladder rupture is nearly always managed by surgery and primary closure of the rent. Dehiscence and rerupture in the few days following surgery are not uncommon, and routine placement of an indwelling urinary catheter for 3 to 5 days after surgery may keep the bladder wall free of tension and challenge to the suture line. Conservative management of bladder ruptures also involves placement of an indwelling catheter and a long-term regimen of antimicrobials and has yielded favorable results.[58] It is tempting to surmise that this approach is most likely to yield success when the rent is not large and when it involves the dorsal aspect of the bladder. This option may be feasible when the owners are not able to finance abdominal surgery, and the bladder rent involves the dorsal wall and is modest in size. Nonsurgical management of bladder rupture in 4 adult horses was recently reported.[59]

Ultrasound imaging can distinguish between other problems affecting the lower urinary tract and resulting in clinical signs that overlap with those of uroperitoneum. Hematoma formation within the bladder, ascribed to tearing of the intra-abdominal portion of the umbilicus, has been reported and is not an uncommon finding.[60] In some instances, however, the resulting thrombus can be large and obstruct urine flow, leading to signs of stranguria in the foal.

Megavesica is another cause of abdominal enlargement and stranguria, but not uroperitoneum, although it is speculated that some cases of bladder rupture occur

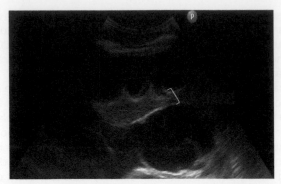

Fig. 19. Sonogram of the right kidney of a foal with renal agenesis. A central band of stroma representing the renal pelvis can be seen (*bracket*), but most of the renal tissue is replaced by anechoic fluid. The foal's left kidney was sonographically normal.

secondary to undetected megavesica.[61,62] Foals with this syndrome of bladder atony and enlargement have been reported, but the cause is not understood. Urine dribbles from the urethra either passively or during straining, and ultrasound reveals a grossly dilated but intact bladder distended with urine.

The kidneys are easily imaged in foals. Renal dysfunction is not unusual in foals, but is usually caused by shock, hypoperfusion, septic injury, and toxicosis from administration of nephrotoxic medications. Congenital renal conditions are uncommon in horses, but polycystic kidney disease and renal agenesis (**Fig. 19**) and renal/glomerular hypoplasia[63,64] are occasionally reported. A recent case report[61] detailed a diffuse, bilateral alteration of renal parenchyma that was histologically characterized as diffuse cystic renal dysplasia in a 9-day-old thoroughbred foal. The morphologic change in the renal parenchyma was detected with ultrasonography and confirmed at necropsy. Kidneys can have an unremarkable sonographic appearance while being in functional failure; clinicopathologic testing should be done as the primary means of determining renal function.

SUMMARY

Sonographic imaging brings a visual component to the information database for a compromised neonatal foal that can be invaluable for confirming or ruling out many of the differential diagnoses that could be causing the observed clinical or clinicopathologic alterations in the foal. Ultrasound equipment has grown more affordable and more portable in the past decade, and equine practitioners can significantly augment the level of patient care they provide by gaining facility with this safe, fast, noninvasive, and highly informative imaging modality.

REFERENCES

1. Barba M, Lepage OM. Diagnostic utility of computed tomography imaging in foals: 10 cases (2008–2010). Equine Vet Educ 2013;25:29–38.
2. Lascola KM, O'Brien RT, Wilkins PA, et al. Qualitative and quantitative interpretation of computed tomography of the lungs in healthy neonatal foals. Am J Vet Res 2013;74:1239–46.
3. Schliewert EC, Lascola KM, O'Brien RT, et al. Comparison of radiographic and computed tomographic images of the lungs in healthy neonatal foals. Am J Vet Res 2015;76:42–52.

4. Pion L, Perkins G, Ainsworth SM, et al. Use of computed tomography to diagnose a Rhodococcus equi mediastinal abscess causing severe respiratory distress in a foal. Equine Vet J 2001;33:523–6.

5. Lascola KM, Joslyn S. Diagnostic Imaging of the Lower Respiratory Tract in Neonatal Foals: Radiography and Computed Tomography. Vet Clin Equine 2015, in press.

6. Fenton MB. The world through a bat's ear. Science 2011;333:528–9.

7. Bates ME, Simmons JA, Zorikov TV. Bats use echo harmonic structure to distinguish their targets from background clutter. Science 2011;333:627–30.

8. Nickel R, Schummer A, Seiferle E. The viscera of the domestic mammals. 2nd rev edition. Berlin: Springer Verlag; 2013. p. 3–6.

9. Schambourg MA, Laverty S, Mullim S, et al. Thoracic trauma in foals: post mortem findings. Equine Vet J 2003;35:78–81.

10. Jean D, Laverty S, Halley J, et al. Thoracic trauma in newborn foals. Equine Vet J 1999;31:149–52.

11. Sprayberry KA, Bain FT, Seahorn TL, et al. 56 Cases of rib fractures in newborn foals hospitalized in a referral center intensive care unit from 1997 to 2001. Proc Am Assoc Equine Pract 2001;47:395–9.

12. Jean D, Picandet V, Macieira S, et al. Detection of rib trauma in newborn foals in an equine critical care unit: a comparison of ultrasonography, radiography, and physical examination. Equine Vet J 2007;39:158–63.

13. Aleman M, Gillis CL, Nieto JE, et al. Ultrasonographic anatomy and biometric analysis of the thoracic and abdominal organs in healthy foals from birth to age 6 months. Equine Vet J 2002;34:649–55.

14. Sanchez LC, Giguere S, Lester GD. Factors associated with survival of neonatal foals with bacteremia and racing performance of surviving thoroughbreds: 423 cases (1982–2007). J Am Vet Med Assoc 2008;233:1446–52.

15. Stewart AJ, Hinchcliff KW, Saville WJ, et al. Actinobacillus sp bacteremia in foals: clinical signs and prognosis. J Vet Intern Med 2002;16:464–71.

16. Freeman L, Paradis MR. Evaluating the effectiveness of equine neonatal care. Vet Med 1992;87:921–6.

17. Marsh PS, Palmer JE. Bacterial isolates from blood and their susceptibility patterns in critically ill foals: 543 cases (1991–1998). J Am Vet Med Assoc 2001; 218:1608–10.

18. Hong CB, Donahue JM, Giles RC, et al. Etiology and pathology of equine placentitis. J Vet Diagn Invest 1993;5:56–63.

19. Ware LB. Pathophysiology of acute lung injury and the acute respiratory distress syndrome. Sem Respir Crit Care Med 2006;27:337–46.

20. Wheeler AP, Bernard GR. Acute lung injury and the acute respiratory distress syndrome: a clinical review. Lancet 2007;369:1553–65.

21. Sande RD, Tucker RL. Radiology of the equine lungs and thorax. In: Rantanen NW, Hauser ML, editors. The diagnosis and treatment of respiratory disease. Proc Dubai Int equine symp. San Diego (CA): Neyenesch Printers Inc; 1997. p. 139–57.

22. Nykamp SG. The equine thorax. In: Thrall DE, editor. Textbook of veterinary diagnostic radiology. 6th edition. St Louis (MO): Elsevier Saunders; 2013. p. 632–48.

23. Dunkel B, Dolente B, Boston RC. Acute lung injury/acute respiratory distress syndrome in 15 foals. Equine Vet J 2005;37:435–40.

24. Dunkel B. Acute lung injury and acute respiratory distress syndrome in foals. Clin Tech Equine Pract 2006;5:127–33.

25. Wilkins PA, Otto CM, Baumgardner MD, et al. Acute lung injury and acute respiratory distress syndromes in veterinary medicine: consensus definitions: The

Dorothy Russell Havemeyer Working Group on ALI and ARDS in Veterinary Medicine. J Vet Emerg Crit Care 2007;17:333–9.

26. Bernard GR, Artigas A, Brigham KL, et al. The American-European consensus conference on ARDS, definitions, mechanisms, relevant outcomes and clinical trial coordination. Am J Respir Crit Care Med 1994;149:818–24.

27. Peek S, Landolt G, Karasin AI, et al. Acute respiratory distress syndrome and fatal interstitial pneumonia associated with equine influenza in a neonatal foal. J Vet Intern Med 2004;18:132–4.

28. Patterson-Kane JC, Carrick JB, Axon JE, et al. The pathology of bronchointerstitial pneumonia in young foals associated with the first outbreak of equine influenza in Australia. Equine Vet J 2008;40:199–203.

29. Porter M, Ramirez P. Equine neonatal thoracic and abdominal ultrasonography. Vet Clin North Am Equine Pract 2005;21:407–29.

30. Magdesian KG. Neonatal foal diarrhea. Vet Clin North Am Equine Pract 2005;21: 295–312.

31. Hollis AR, Wilkins PA, Palmer JE, et al. Bacteremia in equine neonatal diarrhea: a retrospective study (1990–2007). J Vet Intern Med 2008;22:1203–9.

32. Reef VB. Pediatric abdominal ultrasonography. In: Reef BV, editor. Equine diagnostic ultrasound. Philadelphia: WB Saunders Company; 1998. p. 364–403.

33. Abraham M, Reef VB, Sweeney RW, et al. Gastrointestinal ultrasonography of normal Standardbred neonates and frequency of asymptomatic intussusceptions. J Vet Intern Med 2014;28:1580–6.

34. de Solis Navas C, Palmer JE, Boston RC, et al. The importance of ultrasonographic pneumatosis intestinalis in equine neonatal gastrointestinal disease. Equine Vet J 2012;44(Suppl):64–8.

35. MacKinnon MC, Southwood LL, Burke MJ, et al. Colic in equine neonates: 137 cases (2000–2010). J Am Vet Med Assoc 2013;243:1586–90.

36. Bernard WV, Reef VB, Reimer JM, et al. Ultrasonographic diagnosis of small-intestinal intussusception in three foals. J Am Vet Med Assoc 1989;194:395–7.

37. McGladdery AJ. Ultrasonographic diagnosis of intussusception in foals and yearlings. Proc Am Assoc Equine Pract 1996;40:239–40.

38. Busoni V, De Busscher V, Lopez D, et al. Evaluation of a protocol for fast localized abdominal sonography of horses (FLASH) admitted for colic. Vet J 2011;188:77–82.

39. Soundappan SVS, Holland AJA, Cass DT, et al. Diagnostic accuracy of surgeon-performed focused abdominal sonography (FAST) in blunt paediatric trauma. Injury 2005;36:970–5.

40. Boysen SP, Rozanski EA, Tidwell AS, et al. Evaluation of a focused assessment with sonography for trauma protocol to detect free abdominal fluid in dogs involved in motor vehicle accidents. J Am Vet Med Assoc 2004;225:1198–204.

41. Morresey PR. Umbilical problems. Proc Am Assoc Equine Pract 2014;60:18–21.

42. Whitwell KE. Morphology and pathology of the equine umbilical cord. J Reprod Fertil Suppl 1975;(23):599–603.

43. Reef VB, Collatos C. Ultrasonography of umbilical structures in clinically normal foals. Am J Vet Res 1988;49:2143–6.

44. Reef VB, Collatos C, Spencer PA, et al. Clinical, ultrasonographic, and surgical findings in foals with umbilical remnant infections. J Am Vet Med Assoc 1989;195:69–72.

45. Hackett RP. Rupture of the urinary bladder in neonatal foals. Compend Cont Educ Pract Vet 1984;6:S488–91.

46. Robertson JT, Embertson RM. Surgical management of congenital and perinatal abnormalities of the urogenital tract. Vet Clin North Am Equine Pract 1988;4: 359–79.

47. Wilkins PA. Respiratory distress in foals with uroperitoneum: possible mechanisms. Equine Vet Educ 2004;16:293–5.
48. Wong DM, Leger LC, Scarratt WK, et al. Uroperitoneum and pleural effusion in an American Paint filly. Equine Vet Educ 2004;16:290–3.
49. Richardson DW, Kohn CW. Uroperitoneum in the foal. J Am Vet Med Assoc 1983; 182:267–71.
50. Kablack KA, Embertson RM, Bernard WV, et al. Uroperitoneum in the hospitalised equine neonate: retrospective study of 31 cases, 1988–1997. Equine Vet J 2000; 32:505–8.
51. Dunkel B, Palmer JE, Olson KN, et al. Uroperitoneum in 32 foals: influence of intravenous fluid therapy, infection, and sepsis. J Vet Intern Med 2005;19:889–93.
52. Behr MJ, Hackett RP, Bentinck-Smith J, et al. Metabolic abnormalities associated with rupture of the urinary bladder in neonatal foals. J Am Vet Med Assoc 1981; 178:263–6.
53. Lores M, Lofstedt J, Martinson S, et al. Septic peritonitis and uroperitoneum secondary to subclinical omphalitis and concurrent necrotizing cystitis in a colt. Can Vet J 2011;52:888–92.
54. Franklin RP, Ferrell EA. How to perform umbilical sonograms in the neonate. Proc Am Assoc Equine Pract 2002;48:261–5.
55. Hyman SS, Wilkins PA, Palmer JE, et al. Clostridium perfringens urachitis and uroperitoneum in 2 neonatal foals. J Vet Intern Med 2002;16:489–93.
56. Adams SB, Fessler JF. Umbilical cord remnant infections in foals: 16 cases (1975–1985). J Am Vet Med Assoc 1987;190:316–8.
57. Ortega J, Daft B, Assis RA, et al. Infection of the intestinal umbilical remnant in foals by Clostridium sordelli. Vet Pathol 2007;44:269–75.
58. Lavoie JP, Harnagel SH. Nonsurgical management of ruptured urinary bladder in a critically ill foal. J Am Vet Med Assoc 1998;192:1577–80.
59. Peitzmeier MD, McNally TP, Slone DE, et al. Conservative management of cystorrhexis in four adult horses. Equine Vet Educ 2015. http://dx.doi.org/10.1111/eve.12321.
60. Arnold CE, Chaffin KM, Rush BR. Hematuria associated with cystic hematomas in three neonatal foals. J Am Vet Med Assoc 2005;227:778–80.
61. Rijkenhuizen A. Megavesica and bladder rupture in foals. Equine Vet Educ 2012; 24:404–7.
62. Toth T, Liman J, Larsdotter S, et al. Megavesica in a neonatal foal. Equine Vet Educ 2012;24:396–403.
63. Brown CM, Parks AH, Mullaney TP, et al. Bilateral renal dysplasia and hypoplasia in a foal with an imperforate anus. Vet Rec 1988;122:91–2.
64. Medina-Torres CE, Hewson J, Stampfli S, et al. Bilateral diffuse cystic renal dysplasia in a 9-day-old Thoroughbred filly. Can Vet J 2014;55:141–6.

The Equine Neonatal Cardiovascular System in Health and Disease

 CrossMark

Celia M. Marr, BVMS, MVM, PhD

KEYWORDS

- Prenatal to postnatal adaptation • Dysrhythmia • Cardiac trauma • Cardiac infection
- Pericarditis • Congenital cardiac disease • Echocardiography
- Computed tomography

KEY POINTS

- The neonatal foal is in a transitional state from prenatal to postnatal circulation, and cardiac murmurs are common in neonates because of the flow through shunts.
- Dysrhythmias are present in many foals shortly after birth, but these are usually transient and of little clinical significance.
- The neonatal foal is prone to infection and cardiac trauma, both of which may require intensive monitoring and therapy.
- Echocardiography is the main tool used for valuation of the cardiovascular system, although angiography, nuclear scintigraphy, and computed tomography have important roles.
- Congenital disease represents an interesting diagnostic challenge for the neonatologist, but surgical correction is not appropriate for most equids.

 Videos pertaining to the equine neonatal cardiovascular system accompany this article at http://www.vetequine.theclinics.com/

PRENATAL TO POSTNATAL ADAPTATION

During the first few days of life, the foal, like other neonates, is in a state of transition from intrauterine to extrauterine life; this includes adaptation from fetal to neonatal circulation. Fetal hemoglobin has a higher affinity for oxygen than adult hemoglobin allowing diffusion of oxygen to the fetus in the placenta. The oxygenated blood is carried to the fetus by the umbilical vein, ductus venosus, and caudal vena cava. Oxygenated blood entering the right atrium via the caudal vena cava is directed out of the right side toward the left heart to supply the body, and the flow is diverted away from the noninflated lung. To achieve this, blood flows from the right atrium to the left atrium via the foramen ovale,

Funding and competing interests: none to declare.
Rossdales Equine Hospital and Diagnostic Centre, Cotton End Road, Exning, Newmarket, Suffolk, CB8 7NN, UK
E-mail address: celia.marr@rossdales.com

a fenestrated tubular structure connecting the atria. Additionally, a proportion of blood that passes through the right ventricle (RV) to the pulmonary artery (PA) bypasses the lung by flowing through the ductus arteriosus into the aorta, a process that depends on the high vascular resistance within the fetus's noninflated lung.

In the newborn, the resistance in the pulmonary vasculature decreases with the onset of breathing. The pressure in the left atrium increases relative to the pressure in the right atrium decreasing flow in the foramen ovale. The decrease in circulating prostaglandins that accompanies perinatal adaptation allows closure of ductus arteriosus.

The timing of and mechanisms underlying these events have been extensively studied in other species, particularly lambs and babies, but are relatively unexplored in equids. Flow within the ductus arteriosus is visible in young foals[1] and can be visualized through the foramen ovale in some foals for several weeks after birth.[2] Structural studies have shown that obliteration of the foramen ovale occurs over the first few weeks of life.[3] Ductal closure is initially physiologic, because of constriction of the vessels, and subsequently becomes anatomic as closure with muscular elements occurs.[3,4] Perinatal hypoxia can delay or reverse ductal closure, leading to persistent fetal circulation.[5]

CLINICAL FINDINGS IN THE HEALTHY FOAL

Healthy neonates typically have a heart rate of around 80 beats per minute (bpm), with a regular rhythm, pink mucous membranes, and strong arterial pulses palpable at several sites, including the facial, submandibular, axillary, metatarsal, and coccygeal arteries. The heart rate can vary considerably with excitement during veterinary examination. The transition from a prenatal to postnatal pattern of circulation accounts for findings on cardiac auscultation, and cardiac murmurs are very commonly found in healthy equine neonates.[1,6] Flow within the ductus arteriosus creates a machinery murmur high and cranially over the left heart base that usually disappears within the first few days of life.[1] Systolic murmurs are also common in young foals. Some of these may be due to flow through the foramen ovale but some likely relate to flow in the great vessels, the most common cause of physiologic murmurs in adults. The foal's relatively thin body wall means these physiologic murmurs are very easy to detect and they can often be quite loud. In foals with loud murmurs shortly after birth that show no other signs of cardiovascular compromise, it is often appropriate simply to monitor the foal over the next few weeks to ensure that the cardiac murmur becomes less prominent.[1,6] Cardiac disease should be suspected in foals with loud, widely radiating murmurs, particularly if they are associated with a precordial thrill. Foals with heart disease may be stunted or fail to gain weight and have other more specific cardiovascular signs, such as dependent edema, jugular distension and pulsation, pleural effusion, ascites, weakness, and collapse.

CARDIAC DYSRHYTHMIAS IN THE NEONATE

Dysrhythmias are common in the newborn foal. Atrial fibrillation, supraventricular tachycardia, ventricular premature depolarizations, ventricular tachycardia, idioventricular rhythm, and second-degree atrioventricular block have all been documented transiently within 15 minutes of birth.[7] These dysrhythmias are not usually identified in healthy foals except where parturition is closely supervised by a veterinarian; but if they are detected, generally the most appropriate course of action is simply to monitor the rhythm for a few minutes. An electrocardiogram (ECG) is required to characterize the specific rhythm disturbances and antidysrhythmic therapy, if required, should adhere to guidelines available for adults.[8] For sustained, rapid, unstable ventricular tachycardia, appropriate antidysrhythmic drugs include intravenous (IV) quinidine gluconate (0.5–2.2 mg/kg IV every 10 minutes), lignocaine (0.25–0.5 mg/kg IV), and propranolol (0.03–0.1 mg/kg IV). There are no studies critically evaluating the efficacy or potential harms associated with the use of these drugs in neonates or horses in general. The author's preference for first choice for ventricular tachycardia and rapid atrial fibrillation is quinidine gluconate and/or propranolol (**Fig. 1**).

In compromised foals delivered during dystocia, sinus bradycardia progressing to electromechanical dissociation and asystole can occur. Appropriate emergency therapy includes epinephrine (0.005–0.01 mg/kg IV) or atropine (0.005–0.01 mg/kg IV). These drugs often have a relatively transient effect and can produce short periods of very rapid tachycardia. Consideration should be given to transcutaneous pacing that can result in a more stable and effective heart rate. With this technique, electrodes are placed over both sides of the heart. It is important to dry the foal to allow the electrodes to adhere, and the use of an elasticated belt or bandage is helpful in this setting

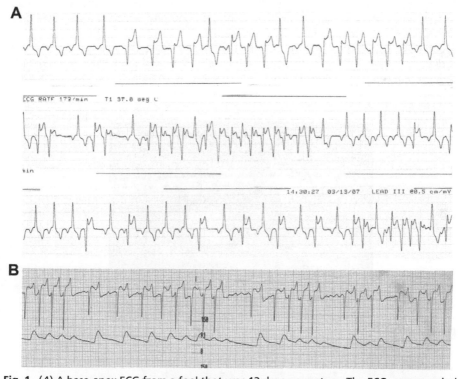

Fig. 1. (*A*) A base-apex ECG from a foal that was 12 days premature. The ECG was recorded shortly after delivery in a terminal caesarian section, which was necessary because the mare had severe orthopedic disease. Rapid, polymorphic ventricular tachycardia is present. This tachycardia resolved in response to IV boluses of quinidine gluconate together with intranasal oxygen and other supportive measures. The foal was euthanized at 27 hours of age because of severe neurologic dysfunction. Paper speed 25 mm/s, 1 mV = 1 cm. (*B*) A base-apex ECG from a 4-week-old foal (87 kg) under general anesthesia in a 4-week-old filly undergoing an attempt to remove a broken catheter fragment from the PA (see later discussion) with a transvenous grasping device. There is rapid atrial fibrillation with complexes of varying size, most likely of supraventricular origin. The direct arterial pressure trace (below ECG) shows the impact of the dysrhythmia on blood pressure. This dysrhythmia resolved with treatment with 2.6 mg propranolol and 48 mg quinidine gluconate IV. Paper speed 25 mm/s, 1 mV = 1 cm.

as the electrodes are easy to dislodge (**Fig. 2**). The desired heart rate is selected (usually around 70–80 bpm), and the current is increased in increments until capture is successful. Relatively low currents are used; therefore, personnel working on the foal are not in any danger, although they may occasionally feel the current (Video 1).

DIAGNOSTIC IMAGING

In comparison with adults, thoracic radiography is much less challenging in foals and provides much more information. In most neonates both lateral and dorsoventral thoracic radiographs can be obtained. Radiography is less sensitive than echocardiography in estimating heart size, but large changes in cardiac dimensions may be apparent; with left-to-right shunting, overcirculation of the pulmonary vasculature may be present. Angiography can be useful in the demonstration of intracardiac and extracardiac shunts.[9] Nuclear angiography is an alternative noninvasive means of demonstrating left-to-right shunts.[10,11] However, as these are complex procedures, they are now used less extensively than echocardiography, which has the great benefits of being noninvasive and widely accessible.

A complete echocardiographic examination involves systematic evaluation of each cardiac structure individually to determine its structure and its position in relation to other structures.[12,13] **Table 1** describes a basic approach to echocardiographic

A

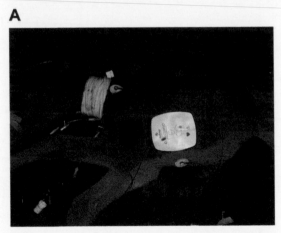

B

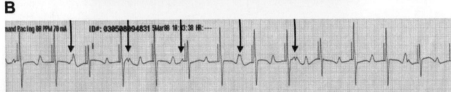

Fig. 2. (*A*) For transcutaneous pacing in a bradycardic neonate during resuscitation following dystocia and transvaginal delivery, electrodes are placed over the heart on the left (*rectangular pad*) and right side. The hair has been clipped and the foal dried. It is also helpful to secure these with an elasticated girth fixed (not shown in this image). Note monitoring electrodes (*circular pads*) are also in place in this foal. (*B*) Delivery of the pacing current is indicated by the vertical lines and these are immediately followed by QRS-T complexes confirming that capture is achieved at a current of 70 mA and a paced ventricular rate of 80 bpm. Arrows indicate P waves occurring independently, and this spontaneous sinus rate is around 50 bpm. Paper speed 25 mm/s, 1 mV = 1 cm.

examination and includes some reference ranges for neonatal thoroughbreds. Additional information on echocardiographic cardiac dimensions in the foals of other breeds is available.[14-16]

Two-dimensional echocardiography allows valve, chamber, and vessel anatomy to be defined. M-mode echocardiography is useful for precise measurement of dimensions, whereas Doppler techniques are used to define intracardiac flow and identify valvular regurgitation and shunts associated with congenital cardiac disease. Contrast echocardiography is particularly applicable in congenital cardiac disease[17,18] and can add to the information obtained from spectral and color flow Doppler echocardiography. Contrast echocardiography involves the administration of a mixture of equal volumes of patients' blood and saline shaken with a small volume of air via the jugular vein. The microbubbles within the solution can be seen as they travel through the heart. With right-to-left shunting, bubbles can be seen entering the left side of the circulation. With left-to-right shunting, or lesions, a negative contrast effect is observed, as anechoic blood is visible within an echogenic chamber.

In healthy neonates, the RV is often relatively large in comparison with the left ventricle (LV) (**Fig. 3**), reflecting the transitional phase from fetal to postnatal circulation. Intraoperator and interoperator variability for most standard measurements of LV size and function is low, but repeated measurements of RV and left atrial appendage diameters should be interpreted with caution because of high variability.[19] Young foals also tend to have low fractional shortening, but otherwise the general principles of interpretation of echocardiographic images differs little from the approach taken in adults.

Both Doppler and volumetric echocardiographic methods are available for noninvasive monitoring of cardiac output.[20] In standing adult horses, the 4-chamber area-length, Simpson, bullet, and Doppler from the RV outflow tract provided best agreement with lithium dilution.[21] Of these, the bullet method is perhaps the least technically challenging and it can readily be performed in the neonatal intensive care unit (see **Fig. 3**; Videos 2 and 3).

CARDIAC CATHETERIZATION AND ESTIMATION OF PULMONARY ARTERY PRESSURE

Cardiac catheterization allows pressure and oxygen tensions to be measured within various chambers to document intracardiac shunting.[22] Catheterization can also be useful to demonstrate pulmonary hypertension in foals with pulmonary disease and involves placement of a Swan-Ganz catheter via the jugular vein. Measurement of the PA diameter is a noninvasive alternative as dilation suggests pulmonary hypertension. The ratio of the right PA in diastole measured in the right parasternal long-axis image of the LV outflow tract to the aortic diameter in the same image is larger in foals with severe pneumonia suggesting this may be a useful indicator of pulmonary hypertension (**Fig. 4**).

CARDIAC DISEASES IN THE NEONATAL PERIOD

Although intuitively one might expect that congenital cardiac disease would be the most common form of cardiac disease seen in the neonatal period, in reality, congenital cardiac disease is fairly uncommon. Furthermore, many foals with congenital cardiac disease cope during the neonatal period but go on to present with signs of cardiovascular compromise at older ages, usually defined by the severity of the specific derangements. Pericardial,[23] myocardial, and endocardial involvement can occur with sepsis, although these sites are less common than others, such as umbilical vessels, joints, and the gastrointestinal and respiratory systems. Trauma to the heart is an important potential sequel to rib fracture and can be iatrogenic.

Table 1
Basic approach to echocardiographic imaging in foals

Image Plane and Imaging Mode	Main Features in Healthy Foals	Specific Lesions to Rule In or Out	Measurements[a]
Right parasternal long-axis with transducer positioned in the fourth intercostal space and aligned at approximately 10° from vertical			
RV outflow view, 2-dimensional and Doppler	Orientating cranially, visualize right atrium, RV, and RV outflow tract; confirm that PA branches	Assess valve and chamber structure and attachments; use to identify pulmonary regurgitation and pulmonary dilation and for placement of spectral Doppler cursor/sample volume for pulmonic outflow	PA diameter diastole = 2.83–3.09 cm
LV outflow view, 2-dimensional and Doppler	Orientating straight across the chest, visualize aorta and parts of the LV and RV and atria; right branch of the PA lies deep to aorta; confirm coronary arteries arise from aorta	Assess valve and chamber structure and attachments; look for ventricular septal defects; use to identify aortic and tricuspid regurgitation and pulmonary dilation; aligning slightly cranially, may see flow from aorta to PA via the ductus arteriosus	Aortic diameter diastole = 2.8–3.05 cm
Four-chamber view, 2-dimensional and Doppler	Orientating slightly caudally, visualize right atrium, RV, left atrium, and LV; note RV is large relative to LV in healthy foals	Assess valve and chamber structure	—
Right parasternal short-axis with transducer positioned in the fourth intercostal space and aligned at approximately 10° from horizontal			
Aortic view, 2-dimensional and M mode	Visualize aorta, aortic valve cusps, PA, and its branches; confirm PA branches and coronary arteries arise from aorta	Assess valve structure and anatomy of great vessels; look for subpulmonic ventricular septal defect. Use to guide M mode cursor placement for aortic M mode and for placement of spectral Doppler cursor/sample volume for pulmonic outflow	—
Mitral valve view, 2-dimensional and M mode	Visualize mitral and tricuspid valve cusps	Assess valve structure; use 2-dimensional image to guide M mode cursor placement for mitral M mode	Distance between the septum and the E point of the mitral valve = 0.39–0.55 cm

View	Description	Assessment	Values[a]
Ventricular view, 2-dimensional and M mode	Visualize LV and RV	Assess chamber structure and size; look for muscular ventricular septal defects; use to 2-dimensional image to guide M mode cursor placement for ventricular M mode	Interventricular septal thickness in diastole = 1.47–1.65 cm; LV internal diameter in diastole = 5.09–5.76 cm; LV free wall thickness in diastole = 1.00–1.19 cm; Interventricular septal thickness in systole = 2.14–2.44 cm; LV internal diameter in systole = 3.35–3.90 cm; LV free wall thickness in systole = 1.55–1.84 cm; Fractional shortening percentage = 29.6–36.4, may be slightly lower in first few days
Left parasternal long-axis			
Left atrial view, 2-dimensional and Doppler	Obtain from fifth intercostal space, orientating roughly vertically; visualize left atrium and LV and caudal vena cava transversely.	Assess valve structure and chamber size; use to identify mitral regurgitation	Left atrial diameter 5.35–6.02 cm
Aortic view, 2-dimensional and Doppler	Obtain from fourth intercostal space, orientating slightly craniodorsally; visualize aortic outflow	Assess valve structure; use to identify aortic regurgitation and for placement of spectral Doppler cursor/sample volume for aortic outflow	—
Pulmonic view, 2-dimensional and Doppler	Obtain from third intercostal space orientating slightly craniodorsally; can image through triceps muscle; visualize PA	Assess valve structure; use to identify pulmonic regurgitation and subjectively assess PA size; look for retrograde flow in PA with patent ductus arteriosus	—

[a] Data represent 95% confidence intervals for healthy thoroughbred foals aged 1 week and weighing 61.7 ± 6.5 kg (mean ± standard deviation). *Data from Ref.[6]*

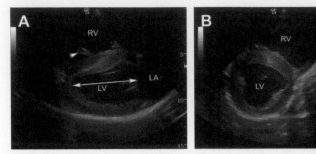

Fig. 3. Right parasternal long- (*A*) and short-axis (*B*) images of the ventricles in a 1-day-old foal. The long-axis image is optimized to show the apical region. The RV is relatively large compared with the LV, which is normal in a neonate. Note the moderator band in the RV (*arrowhead*). For the bullet method of estimating cardiac output (CO), the LV length (*arrow*) is measured from the long-axis image (*A*); the basal area just below the mitral valve is derived from the short-axis image (*B*) at end-systole and end-diastole volume (V). V = 5/6 × basal area × LV length. CO = end-diastole V − end-systolic V × HR. LA, left atrium. For corresponding images see Videos 2 and 3.

CARDIAC TRAUMA

Thoracic trauma is a common event associated with parturition, but it is not always clinically significant.[24] Fillies, primiparous mares, and dystocia are risk factors.[24,25] In foals admitted to one intensive care unit, the prevalence was almost 20%.[25] The left side is affected more than the right, and the most common form of thoracic asymmetry is costochondral dislocation.[24] The most common site of fracture is near the costochondral junction[26]; in this location, the distal part of the rib is typically displaced laterally.[25] Where fractures occur in the midsections, and particularly when multiple ribs are involved, there is potential for medial displacement and intrathoracic trauma leading to hemothorax, lung contusion, or pericardial and myocardial trauma (Video 4). With multiple rib fractures, diaphragmatic trauma and displacement of portions of the gastrointestinal tract into the thorax are possible (Video 5).

Otherwise healthy foals with rib fracture will often remain very bright and relatively asymptomatic, although they may be tachycardic, presumably reflecting pain. Fracture and costochondral dislocation can be suspected based on palpation of thoracic asymmetry, and careful palpation of the symmetry of the chest should be included in the physical examination of all neonates because of the high prevalence of this

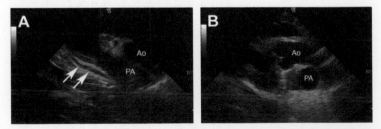

Fig. 4. (*A*) Right parasternal long-axis image of the RV outflow tract from a 43-day-old foal with acute respiratory distress syndrome and Rhodococcal pneumonia. In this image, dilation of the PA is evident, suggesting pulmonary hypertension. There is also a mild pericardial effusion (*arrows*). (*B*) Right parasternal long-axis image of the LV outflow tract from a 43-day-old foal with acute respiratory distress syndrome and rhodococcal pneumonia. The ratio of the diameters of the PA to the aorta (Ao) is 1.01, confirming PA dilation.

problem. Ultrasonography (**Fig. 5**) is more sensitive than radiography for the identification of rib fratures,[25] and it allows the intrathoracic structures to be evaluated carefully (**Fig. 6**, Videos 6 and 7). Computed tomography can be useful in complex cases, particularly for surgical planning (**Fig. 7**).

The management of rib fractures must take account of both the current and potential intrathoracic trauma and the foal's general clinical status. Foals that are compromised (for example, because of neonatal maladjustment syndrome or sepsis) are likely to be recumbent and seem to be more prone to intrathoracic complications. Foals that are otherwise healthy can be managed conservatively with judicious use of analgesics and restricted exercise coupled with frequent and careful ultrasonographic monitoring to detect any intrathoracic trauma. For foals with multiple rib fractures and particularly when the intrathoracic trauma includes cardiac trauma, surgical stabilization of the thoracic cage is indicated. Options include the use of reconstruction plates[27] and a nylon strand suture repair technique[28] (see **Fig. 7**). An inexpensive alternative using nylon cable ties has also been reported.[29]

Foals undergoing therapy that includes the use of intravenous catheters are at risk of iatrogenic cardiac trauma. It is not clear whether there is an increased risk of catheter breakage in foals compared to adults. Foals are often able to scratch the catheter site in their necks in a manner not possible for an adult horse. More likely, the risk of catheter breakage is not influenced by age; but the size of the foal means that the broken catheter fragment becomes lodged within the heart or great vessels, most often in the RV. In larger foals, the catheter may traverse the heart and become lodged in the PA (**Fig. 8**, Videos 8–10). In adults, broken catheter fragments generally travel to the lungs from where they cannot be retrieved; but fortunately complications are unlikely.

Although an early report described a successful outcome following thoracotomy,[30] retrieval of broken catheter fragments using transvenous grasping devices is a more appropriate approach currently.[31,32] In one foal managed by the author, which was 4 weeks old and weighed 87 kg at presentation, the catheter became lodged in the right and main pulmonary arteries (see **Fig. 8**). The foal had mild pneumothorax and pulmonary lesions; therefore, attempts to retrieve this with a snare with 100-cm catheter length and a working diameter of 12 to 20 mm (Merit Medical Standard Snare System, Menlo Park, CA http://infinitimedical.com/products/snare/) failed. The foal

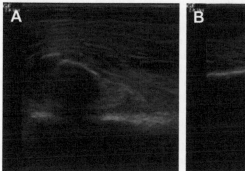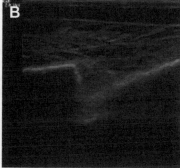

Fig. 5. Transverse (*A*) and longitudinal (*B*) ultrasonography of the left fifth rib in a newborn filly with fractures of the third to the eighth left. This filly had no additional medical problems and had an uneventful outcome with conservative management. The fractures are often easiest to see in the transverse images (*A*) and, once located, the transducer can then be orientated along the long axis (*B*) of the rib to further characterize displacement. In this example, the distal portion (on the left of the image) is displaced laterally; other ribs had distal fragments that were displaced medially.

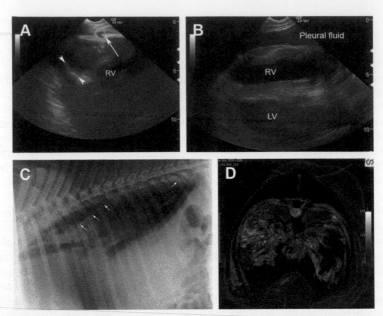

Fig. 6. Ultrasonography, lateral thoracic radiographs, and computed tomography (CT) images from a 4-day-old filly foal that sustained fractures to the left third to ninth ribs. The extent of the damage was not fully appreciated at birth. By day 4, the filly had developed weakness, tachypnea, and anemia, prompting further investigations. (*A*) Large amounts of fluid are visible on either side of the mediastinum (*arrowheads*). One of the fractures is visible (*arrow*) and the end of the dorsal fragment and is surrounded by hemorrhage in an extrathoracic hematoma. Small speckles are visible within the fluid suggesting the presence of air. For corresponding images see Video 6. (*B*) Pleural fluid (hemorrhage) surrounds the heart, but there is minimal evidence of pericardial hemorrhage. These findings helped to determine the decision to manage this filly without surgical stabilization of the ribs. The large number of ribs involved and the duration before assessment were additional factors taken into consideration. After drainage of approximately 3 L of pleural fluid (while whole-blood transfusion was given), the foal's respiratory rate and pattern improved. For corresponding images see Video 7. (*C*) There is pleural effusion and pneumothorax, but it is difficult to discern any rib fractures. The contours of the collapsed lung are shown with arrows. (*D*) A CT subsequently showed further expansion of the pneumothorax. In this 3-dimensional CT reconstruction, focusing on the dorsal two-thirds of the thorax, bilateral pneumothorax is visible, worse on the left than right. Most of the left lung and the ventral portion of the right lung are collapsed. With this color map, the better-aerated portions of the lung are orange-yellow and the abnormal portions are purple and gray. Fragments of ribs are visible (left ribs = right side of image). Note the image plane is slightly oblique such that some of the right lung seems to lie outside the ribs (*artifact*). The pneumothorax was aspirated, and the foal was discharged from the hospital 8 days later.

remained free of clinical signs and was treated for 4 weeks with antimicrobials. Radiographs at that time were unremarkable, and the foal has shown no clinical consequences and remains healthy at 3 years old.

CARDIAC INFECTION

Cardiac involvement in neonatal sepsis can be both direct and indirect. The heart is one of many organs involved in the systemic inflammatory response syndrome that is very commonly encountered. Management of the septic neonate, and those

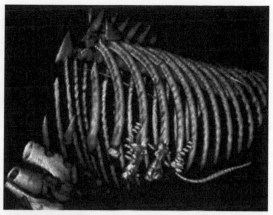

Fig. 7. This filly had 2 ribs stabilized with reconstruction plates (*right* 5 and 6) and 2 stabilized with nylon suture (*right* 4 and 7). There was no intervention for the laterally displaced fracture of the left 6. Additional factors taken into consideration were that the filly had severe neonatal maladjustment syndrome and some abnormalities of conformation. She was recumbent and considered to be at high risk of cardiac trauma. Computed tomography can be helpful for surgical planning.

compromised for other reasons, very often includes careful cardiovascular monitoring and therapies to support blood pressure and cardiac output.

Young horses are at increased risk of infective endocarditis compared with adults; but this condition is not specifically associated with the neonatal age group, perhaps because very young foals are more likely to present with signs of fulminant sepsis affecting multiple organs rather than have colonization of a single or group of heart valves. Primary myocardial dysfunction is difficult to recognize in neonates because echocardiographic indicators are relatively crude and healthy foals often have rather low fractional shortening. A study using the myocardial biomarkers, CK-MB and cardiac troponin, suggested that myocardial injury occurs during septicemia in neonatal foals but that the injury is not associated with survival among septic foals.[33] Blood pressure and cardiac output should be monitored when myocardial injury is suspected; pressors, such as dobutamine, should be used to support cardiac output.

FIBRINOUS PERICARDITIS

Fibrinous pericarditis is an unusual presentation with neonatal sepsis. To date, 4 cases have been reported, one of which was associated with *Actinobacillus equuli*.[34] Affected foals present with clinical signs of right heart dysfunction including ventral edema and jugular pulsation and distension. The heart sounds may be muffled, and echocardiography confirms accumulation of fluid and fibrinous material within the pericardial sac. In adults, successful treatment of fibrinous pericarditis involves broad-spectrum antimicrobials with pericardial drainage and lavage. In the neonates that have been reported to date, a similar approach was not successful; therefore, it seems a guarded prognosis is warranted in neonates with fibrinous pericarditis.[23,34]

CONGENITAL CARDIAC DISEASE

Congenital cardiac defects accounted for 3.5% of all congenital defects in one pathologic survey[35]; but in a species primarily bred[36] and maintained for athletic purposes,

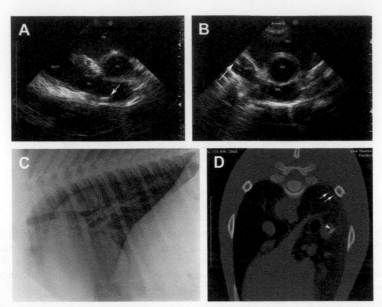

Fig. 8. Ultrasonography, radiographs, and a computed tomography (CT) image from a 4-week-old filly with a broken catheter fragment in her main and right PA. (*A*) In the right parasternal long-axis image of the RV outflow tract (RVOT) the distal end of the catheter is visible in the PA about 3 to 4 cm from the pulmonary valve (*arrow*). For corresponding images see Video 8. (*B*) In the right parasternal short-axis image optimized to view the right PA (RPA), a portion of the catheter fragment is visible (*arrow*). For corresponding images see Video 9. (*C*) Radiographs demonstrate the location of the catheter but do not distinguish left from right PA branches. There are some fluffy multifocal interstitial patterns, particularly dorsal to the catheter tip, suggesting pulmonary disease. (*D*) A CT image showing a section of the catheter in the RPA (*arrowhead*). There is pneumothorax (*arrow*) and evidence of pulmonary pathology in the right lung. For corresponding images see Video 10. Ao, aorta; RA, right atrium.

it is perhaps unsurprising that the prevalence of congenital cardiac disease is lower in horses than in some of the other domestic species. It is estimated to occur in around 1 to 5 in 1000 births[37]; but compared with the prevalence in the author's local thoroughbred population, that estimate seems to be rather high.

The Arabian breed is at particular risk of congenital cardiac disease; but to date no heritability or genomic studies have addressed this issue, although a genetic liability has been shown with atrial fibrillation in the Standardbred breed.[36] Simple ventricular septal defect (VSD) is the most common form of congenital cardiac defect identified in the horse; among the complex defects, tetralogy of Fallot and tricuspid atresia seem to be the most prevalent.[38]

VENTRICULAR SEPTAL DEFECT

VSDs have been documented in a wide variety of breeds, and the lesion is particularly common in Welsh mountain ponies. The defects are usually located in the membranous (nonmuscular) portion of the septum in the LV outflow tract (subaortic) immediately below the right coronary cusp of the aortic valve and the tricuspid valve.[39–41] Less commonly, defects are found in the RV outflow tract (subpulmonic), the perimembranous or muscular portions of the septum where there may be single, multiple, or fenestrated.[42,43] With 2-dimensional echocardiography, a membranous VSD is typically best visualized in an image of the LV outflow tract[39,44] (see **Table 1**). The defect should be measured in 2 mutually perpendicular planes to determine its maximal diameter. Color flow Doppler echocardiography demonstrates the intracardiac shunt and is particularly helpful in identifying small VSDs. Continuous wave Doppler echocardiography is used to document the maximal velocity of the intracardiac shunt: The maximal shunt velocity reflects the pressure difference between the left and RVs. If the RV pressure increases, the pressure difference will decrease; therefore, the shunt velocity will be low (<4 m/s).[39]

Although larger membranous defects can lead to heart failure in the neonatal age group, most patients with simple VSD are at least several weeks old at presentation (except where it is detected on a routine perinatal examination in an otherwise healthy individual). Therefore, if a VSD is detected in a compromised neonate, a careful search for additional lesions should be conducted. With simple defects, the shunt direction is usually left to right; however, with additional lesions, such as bicuspid pulmonary valve, bidirectional shunting may exist.[45]

TETRALOGY OF FALLOT

Tetralogy of Fallot is the most common form of right-to-left shunt seen in foals.[38,46–52] The tetralogy consists of a large VSD, pulmonic stenosis, and overriding of the aorta and RV hypertrophy, whereas the pentalogy has, in addition, an atrial septal defect.[53,54] The right-to-left shunt develops because of pulmonic stenosis; the pressures within the RV exceed those of the LV. This form of shunting creates systemic hypoxemia, tissue hypoxia, cyanosis, exercise intolerance, polycythemia, hypcrviscosity of the blood, and stunting of growth. Foals typically have a loud systolic murmur with its point of maximal intensity over the pulmonary valve on the left side. Echocardiography illustrates the various components of the defect.[52] Most patients die or are euthanized because of the severity of their clinical signs early in life; however, the degree of cardiac compromise depends on the degree of pulmonic stenosis; survival to 3[49] and 7 years of age[51] has been reported.

CRITICAL PULMONIC STENOSIS AND PULMONIC ATRESIA

Knowledge of critical pulmonic stenosis is important for the neonatologist because affected foals are severely compromised from birth.[55] With an extremely stenotic PA, most of the blood flows from the right atrium to the left atrium through the foramen ovale and a left-to-right shunt through the ductus arteriosus supplies the lungs. Affected foals have loud murmurs and are severely hypoxic. There is no increase in arterial oxygen tension following the administration of intranasal oxygen; thus, blood gas analysis is a helpful diagnostic procedure. This finding is similar to that of persistent fetal circulation,[5] and the two conditions must be differentiated by echocardiographic examination. A variation of this defect is atresia of the PA.[56,57] In pulmonic atresia, the RV and PA do not communicate; this can also occur with[58,59] and without VSD.[57] Affected foals are likely to be extremely cyanotic with loud murmurs; they may able to survive in the short-term because of a variety of alternative communications between the PA and the systemic circulation via the descending aorta.[58]

OTHER CONGENITAL CARDIAC DISEASES

There is a range of other complex congenital cardiac abnormalities: Affected foals present early in life with loud widely radiating cardiac murmurs, precordial thrill, and, depending on the specific defect, sometimes cyanosis. These defects can all be differentiated using echocardiography, angiography, computed tomography, and other diagnostic techniques, such as cardiac catheterization.

Sequential segmental analysis is essential for the identification of congenital cardiac disease, particularly derangements or transposition of the great vessels (**Fig. 9**). This analysis involves assessing cardiac structures in a series of steps[13] that allow the clinician to identify the specific defects.

Step 1: Atrial Arrangement

The right has a triangular appendage, and the left is tubular and narrow based. Congenital right atrial diverticulum has been reported,[60] and atrial septal defects can occur in isolation[61,62] or as part of complex conditions.[54]

Step 2: Ventricular Arrangement

The RV has coarse apical trabeculations, leaflet of the atrioventricular valve attached directly to the septum, moderator band, and septomarginal trabeculations; the left has fine trabeculations and smooth upper part of the septum without attachment of the atrioventricular valve. The ventricular morphology can be indeterminate, that is, a solitary ventricle with no ventricular septum.[63,64] Hypoplastic ventricles are complete or incomplete and lack the inlet portion.[61,63,65,66]

Step 3: Atrioventricular Connections

If there are 2 atria, these are either connected to the appropriate ventricle (concordant) or not (discordant). Biatrial, univentricular connections occur where the atria connect to only one ventricle (double[63]) or one atrium ends blindly in a muscular floor at the atrioventricular junction (atrioventricular valve atresia[38,53,67–75]). Usually, the connected ventricle is dominant and the nonconnected ventricle is hypoplastic. Solitary ventricles[76] and uniatrial, biventricular connection can also occur.

Step 4: Atrioventricular Valves

The number of cusps,[64,77] their shape and connections, regurgitation, and stenosis are evaluated.[53,56,64,67–69,72,74,75,78–80]

Step 5: Ventriculo-Arterial Connections

The vessels are identified by their specific features: Coronary arteries originate from the aorta and the main PA branches. If there are 2 great vessels, these are either connected to the appropriate ventricle (concordant) or not (discordant [ie, transposition of the great arteries[73,79,81,82] or double outlet[83,84]]). Vessels may be atretic and difficult or impossible to locate[57] or there may be a single vessel (common arterial trunk[85–88]).

Step 6: Arterial Valves

The number of cusps,[45,89] their shape[90] and connections, regurgitation,[91] and stenosis are evaluated.

Step 7: Associated Malformations

A range of specific lesions should be evaluated and can be classified as follows:

1. Shunts
   a. Atrial,[61] atrioventricular,[64,77] and ventricular septal defects (Ventricular septal defects can occur in isolation[22,38–42,44]; but these defects are also a common

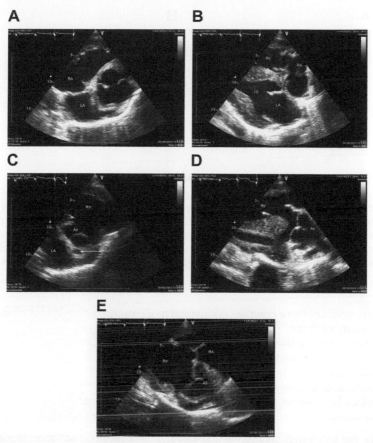

Fig. 9. A series of ultrasonography images from a 4-week-old Suffolk punch filly that demonstrate the sequential segmental approach to the diagnosis of congenital cardiac disease. (*A*) *Step 1 atrial arrangement*: In this short-axis image of the heart base, the left atria (LA) is identified by its narrow appendage and atrial location is correct. It is also apparent that the great vessels are abnormal. (*B*) *Step 2 ventricular arrangement*: In this long-axis 4-chamber image, the ventricles have the correct arrangement but the RV is large compared with the LV. This image also confirms *Step 3 atrioventricular connections*: The relationships between the atria and ventricles are appropriate. *Step 4 the atrioventricular valves* seem to be correctly positioned. (*C–E*) *Step 5 ventriculo-arterial connections*: There is a large vessel from which the coronary arteries (*C, arrow*) are seen to arise in short axis, thus this is the aorta (Ao). Both short (*C*) and long-axis (*D*) show the Ao is connected to the RV. The PA is hard to find; but in a long-axis image of the RV tract area, alongside the Ao, a very small, branching vessel (*E, arrowheads*) can be seen, which is a stenotic PA. *Step 6 arterial valves*: Although not seen clearly in these stills, variations of these 3 images showed that there were 3 aortic cusps. The pulmonic valve cusps could not be visualized clearly. *Step 7 associated malformations* (*1*) *shunts*: a large VSD is visible in the short- (*C*) and long-axis (*D*) images of the midsection of the heart. Together these images confirm double-outlet RV with VSD and pulmonic stenosis. In this foal, a patent ductus arteriosus was also found on postmortem examination but was not demonstrated premortem. RA, right atrium.

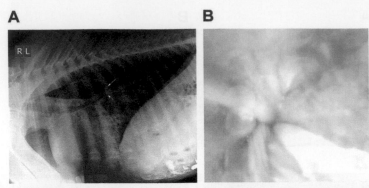

Fig. 10. (*A*) A barium contrast study showing dilation and localized obstruction (*arrows*) of the esophagus in a 2-week-old Welsh mountain pony foal with nasal regurgitation of milk since birth. (*B*) Endoscopy demonstrated that it was possible to insert the endoscopy and reach the stomach and suggested an extramural obstruction. In this image, a plastic tube is used as a guide. Although further studies, such as contrast computed tomography (CT), would have been required to confirm a persistent right aortic arch, this was suspected based on these findings.

component of more complex congenital malformations,[45,53,56,83,92–96] including tetralogy of Fallot.[46–50,52,53])

    b. Patent ductus arteriosus[19,97,98]

    c. Aortopulmonary window[99]

2. Outflow tract obstructions[45,55,100,101]
3. Coronary abnormalities[102]
4. Anomalies of systemic and pulmonary venous connections[103]
5. Abnormalities of the aorta[104,105] and aortic arch[93,106–110]

In foals, the sequential segmental analysis primarily relies on echocardiography; to fully characterize lesions, it is important that the clinician does not overlook alternative imaging modalities, such as radiography (**Fig. 10**) and computed tomography. However, because surgical correction for complex congenital cardiac disease is rarely feasible and cardiac surgery is not a reasonable means of therapy in species primarily used for athletic endeavor, in equids, the need for precise premortem characterization is not pressing and the prognosis for all of the major complex anomalies of the cardiac chambers and great vessels is hopeless.

SUPPLEMENTARY DATA

Supplementary data related to this article can be found online at http://dx.doi.org/10.1016/j.cveq.2015.09.005.

REFERENCES

1. Livesey L, Marr CM, Boswood A, et al. Auscultation and two-dimensional, M mode, spectral and colour flow Doppler echocardiographic findings in pony foals from birth to seven weeks of age. J Vet Intern Med 1998;12:255.
2. Marr CM. Cardiac murmurs: congenital heart disease. In: Marr CM, Bowen IM, editors. Cardiology of the horse. Edinburgh (Scotland): Saunders Elsevier; 2010. p. 193–206.

3. MacDonald A, Fowden AL, Silver M, et al. The foramen ovale of the foetal and neonatal foal. Equine Vet J 1988;20:255–60.
4. Machida N, Yasuda J, Too K, et al. A morphological study on the obliteration processes of the ductus arteriosus in the horse. Equine Vet J 1988;20: 249–54.
5. Cottrill C, O'Connor WN, Cudd T, et al. Persistence of foetal circulatory pathways in a newborn foal. Equine Vet J 1987;19:252–5.
6. Collins NM, Palmer L, Marr CM. Two-dimensional and M-mode echocardiographic findings in healthy thoroughbred foals. Aust Vet J 2010;88:428–33.
7. Yamamoto K, Yasuda J, Too K. Arrhythmias in newborn thoroughbred foals. Equine Vet J 1992;23:169–73.
8. Reef VB, Marr CM. Dysrhythmias: assessment and medical management. In: Marr CM, Bowen IM, editors. Cardiology of the horse. Edinburgh (Scotland): Saunders Elsevier; 2010. p. 159–78.
9. Carlsten J, Kvart C, Jeffcott LB. Method for selective and non-selective angiocardiography in the horse. Equine Vet J 1984;16:47–52.
10. Koblik PD, Hornof WJ. Use of first pass nuclear angiocardiography to detect left-to-right cardiac shunts in the horse. Vet Radiol 1987;28:177–80.
11. Koblik PD, Hornof WJ. Diagnostic radiology and nuclear cardiology. Their use in assessment of equine cardiovascular disease. Vet Clin North Am Equine Pract 1985;1:289–309.
12. Reef VB. Echocardiographic findings in horses with congenital cardiac disease. Comp Contin Educ 1991;13:109–17.
13. Schwarzwald C. Sequential segmental analysis - a systematic approach to the diagnosis of congenital cardiac defects. Equine Vet Educ 2008;20:305–9.
14. Lombard CW, Evans M, Martin L, et al. Blood pressure, electrocardiogram and echocardiogram measurements in the growing pony foal. Equine Vet J 1984;16: 342–7.
15. Stewart J, Rose RJ, Barko A. Echocardiography in foals from birth to three months old. Equine Vet J 1984;16:332–41.
16. Rovira S, Munoz A, Rodilla V. Allometric scaling of echocardiographic measurements in healthy Spanish foals with different body weight. Res Vet Sci 2009;86: 325–31.
17. Bonagura JD, Pipers FS. Diagnosis of cardiac lesions by contrast echocardiography. J Am Vet Med Assoc 1983;182:396–402.
18. Kvart C, Carlsten J, Jeffcott LB, et al. Diagnostic value of contrast echocardiography in the horse. Equine Vet J 1985;17:357–60.
19. Hare TA. A patent ductus arteriosus in an aged horse. J Pathol Bacteriol 1931; 84:124.
20. Lopez L, Colan SD, Frommelt PC, et al. Recommendations for quantification methods during the performance of a pediatric echocardiogram' a report from the Pediatric Measurements Writing Group of the American Society of Echocardiography Pediatric and Congenital Heart Disease Council. J Am Soc Echocardiogr 2010;23:465–95.
21. McConachie E, Barton MH, Rapoport G, et al. Doppler and volumetric echocardiographic methods for cardiac output measurement in standing adult horses. J Vet Intern Med 2013;27:324–30.
22. Critchley KL. The importance of blood gas measurement in the diagnosis of an interventricular septal defect in a horse. A case report. Equine Vet J 1976;8:120–9.
23. Armstrong SK, Raidal SL, Hughes KJ. Fibrinous pericarditis and pericardial effusion in three neonatal foals. Aust Vet J 2014;92:392–9.

24. Jean D, Laverty S, Halley J, et al. Thoracic trauma in newborn foals. Equine Vet J 1999;31:149–52.

25. Jean D, Picandet V, Macieira S, et al. Detection of rib trauma in newborn foals in an equine critical care unit: a comparison of ultrasonography, radiography and physical examination. Equine Vet J 2007;39:158–63.

26. Schambourg MA, Laverty S, Mullim S, et al. Thoracic trauma in foals: post mortem findings. Equine Vet J 2003;35:78–81.

27. Bellezzo F, Hunt RJ, Provost R, et al. Surgical repair of rib fractures in 14 neonatal foals: case selection, surgical technique and results. Equine Vet J 2004;36:557–62.

28. Kraus BM, Richardson DW, Sheridan G, et al. Multiple rib fracture in a neonatal foal using a nylon strand suture repair technique. Vet Surg 2005;34:399–404.

29. Downs C, Rodgerson D. The use of nylon cable ties to repair rib fractures in neonatal foals. Can Vet J 2011;52:307–9.

30. Lees MJ, Read RA, Klein KT, et al. Surgical retrieval of a broken jugular catheter from the right ventricle of a foal. Equine Vet J 1989;21:384–7.

31. Ames TR, Hunter DW, Caywood DD. Percutaneous transvenous removal of a broken jugular catheter from the right ventricle of a foal. Equine Vet J 1991; 23:392–3.

32. Hoskinson JJ, Wooten P, Evans R. Nonsurgical removal of a catheter embolus from the heart of a foal. J Am Vet Med Assoc 1991;199:233–5.

33. Slack JA, McGuirk SM, Erb HN, et al. Biochemical markers of cardiac injury in normal, surviving septic, or nonsurviving septic neonatal foals. J Vet Intern Med 2005;19:577–80.

34. Alcott CJ, Howard J, Wong D, et al. Fibrinous pericarditis and cardiac tamponade in a 3-week-old pony foal. Equine Vet Educ 2013;25:328–33.

35. Crowe MW, Swerczek TW. Equine congenital defects. Am J Vet Res 1984;46: 353–8.

36. Physick-Sheard P, Kraus M, Basrur P, et al. Breed predisposition and heritability of atrial fibrillation in the Standardbred horse: a retrospective case-control study. J Vet Cardiol 2014;16:173–84.

37. Buergelt CD. Equine cardiovascular pathology: an overview. Anim Health Res Rev 2003;4:109–29.

38. Hall TL, Magdesian KG, Kittleson MD. Congenital cardiac defects in neonatal foals: 18 cases (1992-2007). J Vet Intern Med 2010;24:206–12.

39. Reef VB. Evaluation of ventricular septal defect in horses using two-dimensional and Doppler echocardiography. Equine Vet J 1995;(Suppl 19):86–95.

40. Glazier DB, Farrelly BT, O'Connor J. Ventricular septal defect in a 7-year-old gelding. J Am Vet Med Assoc 1975;167:49–50.

41. Lombard C, Scarratt WK, Buergelt CD. Ventricular septal defects in the horse. J Am Vet Med Assoc 1983;167:562–5.

42. Ueno Y, Tomioka Y, Kaneko M. Muscular ventricular septal defect in a horse. Bull Equine Res Inst 1992;29:15–9.

43. Deniau V, Delecroix A. A case of interventricular communication in a racehorse. Practique Veterinaire Equine 2004;36:25–31.

44. Pipers FS, Reef VB, Wilson J. Echocardiographic detection of ventricular septal defects in large animals. J Am Vet Med Assoc 1985;187:810–6.

45. Critchley KL. An interventricular septal defect, pulmonary stenosis and bicuspid pulmonary valve in a Welsh pony foal. Equine Vet J 1976;8:176–8.

46. Prickett ME, Reeves JT, Zent WW. Tetralogy of Fallot in a thoroughbred foal. J Am Vet Med Assoc 1973;162:552–5.

47. Reynolds DJ, Nicholl TK. Tetralogy of Fallot and cranial mesenteric arteritis in a foal. Equine Vet J 1978;10:185–7.
48. Keith J. Tetralogy of Fallot in a quarter horse foal. Vet Med Small Anim Clin 1981; 76:889–95.
49. Cargille J, Lombard C, Wilson JH, et al. Tetralogy of Fallot and segmental uterine dysplasia in a three-year-old Morgan filly. Cornell Vet 1991;81:411–8.
50. Houe H, Koch J, Bindseil E. Tetralogy of Fallot in horses. Dansk Veterinaertidsskrift 1996;79:43–5.
51. Gesell S, Brandes K. Tetralogy of Fallot in a 7-year-old gelding. Pferdeheikunde 2006;22:427–30.
52. Schmitz R, Klaus C, Grabner A. Detailed echocardiographic findings in a newborn foal with tetralogy of Fallot. Equine Vet Educ 2008;20:298–303.
53. Bayly WM, Reed SM, Leathers CW, et al. Multiple congenital heart anomalies in five Arabian foals. J Am Vet Med Assoc 1982;181:684–9.
54. Rahal C, Collatos C, Solano M, et al. Pentalogy of Fallot, renal infarction and renal abscess in a mare. J Equine Vet Sci 1997;17:604–7.
55. Hinchcliff KW, Adams WM. Critical pulmonary stenosis in a newborn foal. Equine Vet J 1991;23:318–20.
56. Meurs KM, Miller MW, Hanson C, et al. Tricuspid valve atresia with main pulmonary artery atresia in an Arabian foal. Equine Vet J 1997;29:160–2.
57. Young LE, Blunden AS, Bartram DH, et al. Pulmonary atresia with an intact ventricular septum in a thoroughbred foal. Equine Vet Educ 1997;9:123–7.
58. Anderson R. The pathological spectrum of pulmonary atresia. Equine Vet Educ 1997;9:128–32.
59. Vitums A, Bayly WM. Pulmonary atresia with dextroposition of the aorta and ventricular septal defect in three Arabian foals. Vet Pathol 1982;19:160–8.
60. Patterson-Kane JC, Harrison LR. Giant right atrial diverticulum in a foal. J Vet Diagn Invest 2002;14:335–7.
61. Physick-Sheard PW, Maxie MG, Palmer NC, et al. Atrial septal defect of the persistent ostium primum type with hypoplastic right ventricle in a Welsh pony foal. Can J Comp Med 1985;49:429–33.
62. Taylor FG, Wotton PR, Hillyer MH, et al. Atrial septal defect and atrial fibrillation in a foal. Vet Rec 1991;128:80–1.
63. Sedacca CD, Bright JM, Boon J. Doppler echocardiographic description of double-inlet left ventricle in an Arabian horse. J Vet Cardiol 2010;12: 147–53.
64. Kraus MS, Pariaut R, Alcaraz A, et al. Complete atrioventricular canal defect in a foal: clinical and pathological features. J Vet Cardiol 2005;7:59–64.
65. Tadmor A, Fischel R, Tov AS. A condition resembling hypoplastic left heart syndrome in a foal. Equine Vet J 1983;15:175–7.
66. Musselman EE, LoGuidice RJ. Hypoplastic left ventricular syndrome in a foal. J Am Vet Med Assoc 1984;185:542–3.
67. Gumbrell RC. Atresia of the tricuspid valve in a foal. N Z Vet J 1970;18:253–6.
68. Button C, Gross DR, Allert JA, et al. Tricuspid atresia in a foal. J Am Vet Med Assoc 1978;172:825–30.
69. van der Linde-Sipman JS, van den Ingh TS. Tricuspid atresia in a foal and a lamb. Zentralbl Veterinarmed A 1979;26A:239–42.
70. Hadlow WJ, Ward JK. Atresia of the right atrioventricular orifice in an Arabian foal. Vet Pathol 1980;17:622–6.
71. Wilson RB, Haffner JC. Right atrioventricular atresia and ventricular septal defect in a foal. Cornell Vet 1987;77:187–91.

72. Honnas C, Puckett MJ, Schumacher J. Tricuspid atresia in a quarter horse foal. Southwest Vet 1987;38:17–20.
73. Zamora CS, Vitums A, Nyrop KA, et al. Atresia of the right atrioventricular orifice with complete transposition of the great arteries in a horse. Anat Histol Embryol 1989;18:177–82.
74. van Nie CJ, van der Kamp JS. Congenital tricuspid atresia in a premature foal (author's transl). Tijdschr Diergeneeskd 1979;104:411–6 [in Dutch].
75. Reef VB, Mann PC, Orsini PG. Echocardiographic detection of tricuspid atresia in two foals. J Am Vet Med Assoc 1987;191:225–8.
76. Zamora CS, Vitums A, Foreman JH, et al. Common ventricle with separate pulmonary outflow chamber in a horse. J Am Vet Med Assoc 1985;186:1210–3.
77. Kutasi O, Voros K, Biksi I, et al. Common atrioventricular canal in a newborn foal–case report and review of the literature. Acta Vet Hung 2007;55:51–65.
78. McGurrin MK, Physick-Sheard PW, Southorn E. Parachute left atrioventricular valve causing stenosis and regurgitation in a thoroughbred foal. J Vet Intern Med 2003;17:579–82.
79. McClure JJ, Gaber CE, Watters JW, et al. Complete transposition of the great arteries with ventricular septal defect and pulmonary stenosis in a thoroughbred foal. Equine Vet J 1983;15:377–80.
80. Duz M, Philbey AW, Hughes KJ. Mitral valve and tricuspid valve dysplasia in a 9-week-old Standardbred colt. Equine Vet Educ 2013;25:339–44.
81. Vitums A, Grant BD, Stone EC, et al. Transposition of the aorta and atresia of the pulmonary trunk in a horse. Cornell Vet 1973;63:41–57.
82. Sleeper MM, Palmer JE. Echocardiographic diagnosis of transposition of the great arteries in a neonatal foal. Vet Radiol Ultrasound 2005;46:259–62.
83. Chaffin MK, Miller MW, Morris EL. Double outlet right ventricle and other associated congenital cardiac anomalies in an American miniature horse foal. Equine Vet J 1992;24:402–6.
84. Fennell L, Church S, Tyrell D, et al. Double-outlet right ventricle in a 10-month-old Friesian filly. Aust Vet J 2009;87:204–9.
85. Rang H, Hurtienne H. Persistent truncus arteriosus in a 2-year old horse. Tierarztl Prax 1976;4:55–8 [in German].
86. Steyn PF, Holland P, Hoffman J. The angiocardiographic diagnosis of a persistent truncus arteriosus in a foal. J S Afr Vet Assoc 1989;60:106–8.
87. Stephen J, Abbott J, Middleton DM, et al. Persistent truncus arteriosus in a Bashkir curly foal. Equine Vet Educ 2000;12:251–5.
88. Jesty SA, Wilkins PA, Palmer JE, et al. Persistent truncus arteriosus in two Standardbred foals. Equine Vet Educ 2007;19:307–11.
89. Michlik KM, Biazik AK, Henklewski RZ, et al. Quadricuspid aortic valve and a ventricular septal defect in a horse. BMC Vet Res 2014;10:142.
90. Taylor SE, Else RW, Keen JA. Congenital aortic valve dysplasia in a Clydesdale foal. Equine Vet Educ 2007;19:4630468.
91. Gross DR, Clark DR, McDonald DR, et al. Congestive heart failure associated with congenital aortic valvular insufficiency in a horse. Southwest. Vet 1977;30:27–34.
92. Muylle E, De Roose P, Oyaert W, et al. An interventricular septal defect and a tricuspid valve insufficiency in a trotter mare. Equine Vet J 1974;6:174–6.
93. van der Linde-Sipman JS, Goedegebuure SA, Kroneman J. Persistent right aortic arch associated with a persistent left ductus arteriosus and an interventricular septal defect in a horse. Tijdschr Diergeneeskd 1979;104(Suppl 4):189–94.

94. Reppas GP, Canfield PJ, Hartley WJ, et al. Multiple congenital cardiac anomalies and idiopathic thoracic aortitis in a horse. Vet Rec 1996;138:14-6.
95. Vitums A. Origin of the aorta and pulmonary trunk from the right ventricle in a horse. Pathol Vet 1970;7:482-91.
96. Rooney GP, Franks WC. Congenital cardiac anomalies in horses. Pathol Vet 1964;1:454-64.
97. Buergelt C, Carmichael JA, Tashjian RJ, et al. Spontaneous rupture of the left pulmonary artery in a horse with patent ductus arteriosus. J Am Vet Med Assoc 1970;186:1210-3.
98. Guarda HI, Schifferlis RCA, Alvarez MLH, et al. A patent ductus arteriosus in a foal. Wiener Tieraztliche Monatsschrift 2005;92:233-7.
99. Valdes-Martinez A, Eades SC, Strickland KN, et al. Echocardiographic evidence of an aortico-pulmonary septal defect in a 4-day-old thoroughbred foal. Vet Radiol Ultrasound 2006;47:87-9.
100. King JM, Flint TJ, Anderson WI. Incomplete subaortic stenotic rings in domestic animals–a newly described congenital anomaly. Cornell Vet 1988;78:263-71.
101. Gehlen H, Bubeck K, Stadler P. Valvular pulmonic stenosis with normal aortic root and intact ventricular and atrial septa in an Arabian horse. Equine Vet Educ 2001;13:286-8.
102. Karlstam E, Ho SY, Shokrai A, et al. Anomalous aortic origin of the left coronary artery in a horse. Equine Vet J 1998;31:350-2.
103. Seco Diaz O, Desrochers A, Hoffmann V, et al. Total anomalous pulmonary venous connection in a foal. Vet Radiol Ultrasound 2005;46:83-5.
104. Amend J, Ross JN, GArner HE, et al. Systolic time intervals in domestic ponies: alterations in a case of coarctation of the aorta. Can J Comp Med 1975;39:62-6.
105. Reimer JM, Marr CM, Reef VB, et al. Aortic origin of the right pulmonary artery and patent ductus arteriosus in a pony foal with pulmonary hypertension and right sided heart failure. Equine Vet J 1993;25:466-70.
106. Bauer S, Livesey MA, Bjorling DE, et al. Computed tomography assisted surgical correction of persistent right aortic arch in a neonatal foal. Equine Vet Educ 2006;18:32-6.
107. Coleman MC, Norman TE, Wall CR. What is your diagnosis? Persistent right aortic arch. J Am Vet Med Assoc 2014;244:1253-5.
108. Scott E, Chaffee A, Eyster GE, et al. Interruption of the aortic arch in two foals. J Am Vet Med Assoc 1978;172:347-50.
109. Bartels JE, Vaughan JT. Persistent right aortic arch in the horse. J Am Vet Med Assoc 1969;154:406-9.
110. Viljoen A, Saulez MN, Steyl J. Right subclavian artery anomaly in an adult Friesian horse. Equine Vet Educ 2012;24:62-5.

Anesthesia of the Equine Neonate in Health and Disease

Berit Fischer, DVM[a],*, Stuart Clark-Price, DVM, MS[b]

KEYWORDS

- Neonate • Foal • Anesthesia • Sepsis • Hyperkalemia • Hypotension
- Hypoventilation • Monitoring

KEY POINTS

- Neonatal foals are different physiologically from adults, resulting in altered pharmacokinetics and pharmacodynamics of anesthetic drugs.
- Performing anesthesia in the neonatal foal requires attentive monitoring of anesthetic depth, circulation, oxygenation, and ventilation because rapid changes needing intervention are common.
- Pain pathways are mature at birth, necessitating appropriate administration of analgesics for invasive procedures.
- The sick neonate frequently has electrolyte, acid–base, and other biochemical derangements that can complicate anesthetic management.
- Specific research targeting anesthesia in the neonatal foal is lacking, and extrapolation of adult equine information should be done with caution.

INTRODUCTION

To induce anesthesia is to provide unconsciousness, analgesia, and muscle relaxation in an individual for the purposes of performing procedures that may otherwise create undo physical and/or psychological stress. Despite these good intentions, anesthetic drugs often have adverse physiologic effects that can lead to increased risk of morbidity and mortality. The equine neonate is particularly susceptible to these adverse effects owing to immaturity of body systems and altered pharmacokinetics and pharmacodynamics of anesthetic drugs with those less than 1 month of age carrying the greatest risk.[1] Understanding the physiologic differences of the neonate

[a] Department of Anesthesia and Pain Management, Animal Medical Center, 510 E. 62 St, New York, NY 10065, USA; [b] Anesthesia and Pain Management, Department of Veterinary Clinical Medicine, College of Veterinary Medicine, University of Illinois, 1008 West Hazelwood Drive, MC-004, Urbana, IL 61802, USA
* Corresponding author.
E-mail address: berit.fischer@amcny.org

Vet Clin Equine 31 (2015) 567–585
http://dx.doi.org/10.1016/j.cveq.2015.09.002
0749-0739/15/$ – see front matter © 2015 Elsevier Inc. All rights reserved.

vetequine.theclinics.com

versus their adult counterparts as well as obstacles that can arise both in the healthy and sick neonate allows the anesthetist to meet the additional challenges these patients pose through better preparation, monitoring, and anesthetic drug administration.

PHYSIOLOGY OF THE NEONATE

Neonates are not small adults. As a whole, neonates have the highest incidence of adverse events and the greatest risk of mortality from anesthesia.[1,2] Their transition to the extrauterine environment results in several rapid changes in organ physiology that require a period of weeks to months to mature. This leaves the neonate in a state of vulnerability when undergoing anesthesia because they are less well-equipped to handle changes in homeostasis. It is important for the anesthetist to be aware of these physiologic differences because they can impact significantly anesthetic management.

The cardiac index is the relationship of cardiac output to body surface area and in the foal, this value is 2- to 3-fold higher than that of an adult and working close to maximal capacity.[3] Unlike the adult horse, the neonatal heart is poorly compliant with limited ability to increase myocardial contractility, resulting in a fixed stroke volume with cardiac output heavily reliant on heart rate. Poor cardiac reflexes, an immature sympathetic nervous system, and a decreased response to catecholamines minimize the ability of the neonate to compensate for hemodynamic changes while under anesthesia, increasing the risk of poor perfusion and inadequate tissue oxygen delivery.[2]

Neonatal foals are also at greater risk for hypoxemia and hypoventilation under anesthesia owing to immature respiratory centers in the brain, decreased functional residual capacity, and an increased metabolic oxygen consumption rate. High minute ventilation allows for rapid changes in the depth of anesthesia and can increase the potential for anesthetic overdose.[4]

Immaturity of the renal, hepatic, and neurologic systems can impact anesthesia in the neonate by potentially increasing the pharmacologic effects of anesthetic drugs. This is the result of a more permeable blood–brain barrier, low albumin levels subsequently leading to decreased drug binding of heavily protein-bound drugs, and decreased hepatic enzyme activity and glomerular filtration rate, resulting in prolonged drug metabolism and excretion.[4,5] Immature liver and kidney also result in impaired gluconeogenesis and glycogenolysis, as well as a decreased ability to tolerate large fluid volumes thus increasing the risk of hypoglycemia and fluid overload.

COMMON REASONS FOR ANESTHESIA

Although placing a neonate under anesthesia should not be taken lightly, there are times when it is necessary. Nonemergent reasons for anesthesia in the neonate are often related to congenital abnormalities, such as angular limb deformities, cleft palate, nonstrangulating hernias, or brachygnathism where correction early in life can lead to a better outcome.

In less fortunate circumstances, neonatal foals may require anesthesia for life-threatening situations such as a ruptured bladder, septic arthritis, trauma, or a gastrointestinal emergency (meconium impaction, small intestinal volvulus, etc). Anesthesia in this subpopulation can carry considerably more risk because these patients tend to have other comorbidities, such as dehydration, sepsis, acid–base and electrolyte abnormalities, and pulmonary dysfunction.

Sedation may suffice for some noninvasive procedures such as catheter placement; however, procedures such as computed tomography or MRI often necessitate general anesthesia to prevent movement, reduce stress, and prevent a potentially dangerous environment for both the patient and personnel. Anesthesia for these procedures should be carried out with the same respect and attention to detail as other more invasive procedures.

PREOPERATIVE EVALUATION

Assessment of the equine neonate for suitability for general anesthesia is similar to the process for other species. A thorough examination of the medical history is necessary to identify all medications and comorbidities because sick neonatal foals frequently are administered multiple medications and have wide-ranging medical problems. A complete physical examination should be performed with a special focus on the cardiovascular, pulmonary, and neurologic systems for identification of specific problems that may impact anesthetic care. Clinical pathology data including a complete blood count, biochemistry panel, and electrolyte and arterial blood gas analysis can provide additional and valuable information about specific disease processes and organ system function. It is important to remember that neonatal foals have an immature metabolic ability, decreased sympathetic nervous tone with a resulting lower systemic blood pressure, increased permeability of the blood–brain barrier, a higher risk and sensitivity to hypothermia, and an increased sensitivity to anesthetic drugs compared with older foals.[5] and should be considered when designing an anesthetic plan. Pulmonary disease is a frequent comorbidity in neonatal foals and imaging studies including computed tomography may be necessary to assess severity.[6,7] Foals with gastrointestinal illness may benefit from abdominal ultrasonography or radiographic examination for anesthetic and surgical planning.

Stabilization before anesthesia is paramount for increasing the odds of a successful outcome. Correction of electrolyte, glycemic, and fluid imbalances are a must and special attention should be given to serum potassium concentrations in foals with urinary tract disease or severe muscle injury because liberation of potassium can be deadly, particularly during anesthesia when changes in pH can occur rapidly. As a rule of thumb, for nonemergent cases a potassium concentration of less than 5.5 mmol/L and, for emergent cases a potassium concentration of less than 6.0 mmol/L should be obtained before anesthesia. Foals requiring insufflation of oxygen while awake for support of blood oxygen content should remain on oxygen through the induction period until intubated and placed on an anesthesia machine. Foals that do not require oxygen support should receive "preoxygenation" with oxygen delivered via an open mask from an anesthesia machine for at least 5 minutes before induction. This increases the time to desaturation and give the anesthetist a cushion of several minutes to allow for more time to intubate the foal.[8]

PHARMACOLOGY
Sedatives and Tranquilizers

Sedatives and tranquilizers can be used for improvement and facilitation of anesthesia in the neonatal foal through calming the patient, easing handling and stress, facilitating catheterization, reducing anesthetic drug dosages, and providing for a smoother induction and recovery. Sedatives and tranquilizers commonly used in equine patients include alpha-2 agonists, benzodiazepines, and phenothiazines.

Alpha-2 agonists such as xylazine, detomidine, and romifidine are favored sedative agents for equine practitioners because of the reliability of sedation when used. These drugs have a mechanism of action through agonism of alpha-2 receptors and a subsequent decrease in the release of neurotransmitters in the brainstem and thus sedation ensues. However, they have the potential for potent adverse cardiopulmonary effects through peripheral alpha receptor agonism that render them less suitable for routine use in neonatal animals. Adverse effects include bradycardia, hypertension, hypotension, upper airway obstruction, decreased minute volume, ataxla, and recumbency.[9] As can be expected, a decrease in cardiac output and cardiac performance occurs during the use of alpha-2 agonists and their use should be minimized in neonatal foals. Additionally, alpha-2 agonist drugs cause a decrease in the motility and blood flow of the gastrointestinal tract and increase urine production and loss of sodium and potassium through antagonism of vasopressin in the renal collecting ducts.[10–13] These adverse effects can be even more magnified in the face of dehydration, sepsis, or hypoxic ischemic encephalopathy.

Benzodiazepines are a particularly useful class of sedative in neonatal foals. Although considered mild and unreliable sedatives in adult horses, in foals less than 2 weeks of age, they can be profoundly sedating. Benzodiazepines are also useful for treatment of seizures and can be administered as a constant rate infusion for prolonged seizure control. Midazolam and diazepam are the most frequently used benzodiazepines in horses and they have similar pharmacokinetic and pharmacodynamic profiles. The mechanism of action of benzodiazepines is through enhancing the action of gamma-aminobutyric acid, a major inhibitory neurotransmitter of the central nervous system. Of the two, midazolam tends to be preferred because of its solubility profile. Diazepam is not soluble in an aqueous solution and thus needs propylene glycol as a vehicle for injection. Propylene glycol is generally considered safe; however, when used in high doses or for prolonged periods, toxic effects can occur, including hyperosmolarity, hemolysis, cardiac arrhythmia, seizures, and lactic acidosis and tissue irritation when administered subcutaneously or intramuscularly.[14] Midazolam is water soluble and thus does not contain propylene glycol in it formulation. Therefore, it can be administered by routes other than intravenously (IV). The pharmacokinetics of midazolam have been described in healthy adult horses but not in foals.[15] Of particular interest for neonatal foals, midazolam decreases the innate immune response of macrophages and neutrophils by suppressing phagocytosis and oxidative burst.[16] However, it is unknown whether this effect is important clinically and it is likely that many other medications commonly used in neonatal foals impact immune function.

The phenothiazine, acepromazine, is a widely used sedative for horses in veterinary medicine. The sedative effects of ace promazine occur through central blockade of dopaminergic receptors. However, ace promazine also causes blockade of peripheral alpha receptors resulting in significant vasodilation and hypotension that can be particularly difficult to treat.[17] The duration of action of ace promazine is dose dependent, but generally lasts for greater than 1 to 2 hours. Additionally, ace promazine also has significant hematologic effects including decreased packed cell volume and reduction in the ability of platelets to aggregate. For these reasons, ace promazine is not particularly useful as a sedative in neonatal foals and should probably be avoided.

Analgesics

Analgesic medications play an important role during recovery from illness of the equine neonate and should not be withheld. It is well-recognized that neonatal animals and humans possess mature pain pathways in the central nervous system, and like in adults, have improved outcomes after surgical procedures when appropriate pain management is employed.[18-21] The most common analgesic options include systemic administration of opioids and nonsteroidal antiinflammatory drugs (NSAID) and regional use of opioids and local anesthetics.

Opioid medications (narcotics) can be classified based on their receptor profiles and generally fall into 4 categories: pure μ agonists, partial μ agonists, agonist–antagonists, and pure antagonists. The pure μ agonists have the greatest ability for pain suppression because, theoretically, there is no ceiling to their analgesic effects. However, questions remain as to their efficacy in adult horses and the potential for adverse effects including decreased intestinal motility, bradycardia, tachycardia, hypoventilation, and excitement.[22,23] However, in foals the opioid fentanyl seems to be well-tolerated and results in dose-dependent sedation.[24,25] Butorphanol, an agonist–antagonist, is among the most commonly used opioids in horses; however, other opioids such as buprenorphine, a partial μ agonist, may be more effective for pain management.[26,27] Butorphanol has been evaluated in healthy foals and seems to be safe when administered IV or intramuscularly. Side effects include sedation and increased feeding behavior[28] and a dose of 0.1 mg/kg but not 0.05 mg/kg provides some analgesia.[29] There are few data available on the pharmacokinetics and pharmacodynamics on the use of pure μ agonist opioids in neonatal foals. In foals with septic arthritis, the clinical impression is that intraarticular preservative-free morphine provides analgesia and in adult horses is shown to be analgesic and has antiinflammatory properties.[30,31]

NSAIDs continue to be a mainstay for analgesia in equine patients. NSAIDs work through either reversible or irreversible suppression of the cyclooxygenase pathway of inflammatory mediator production. Phenylbutazone, flunixin meglumine, meloxicam, firocoxib, aspirin, and carprofen have been used for pain management in foals. The use of NSAIDs in foals must be done with caution because of narrow therapeutic margins and toxicities and adverse effects that can have severe detrimental effects on health. Additionally, practitioners should be cautions when using NSAIDs in foals because of potential differences in pharmacokinetics compared with adult horses. For example, phenylbutazone has a greater volume of distribution, longer half-life, and lesser clearance in foals compared with adult horses.[32] Similarly, flunizim meglumine disposition is different in neonatal foals compared with older foals and the dose and interval may need to be adjusted.[33] Organ systems at particularly high risk of NSAID toxicity include the gastrointestinal, renal, and hepatic systems. Meloxicam (0.6 mg/kg orally every 12 hours) in healthy foals less than 6 weeks of age and firocoxib (0.1 mg/kg orally every 24 hours) in healthy foals less than 2 weeks of age did not demonstrate any immediate clinical adverse effects.[34,35] It is important to remember that pharmacokinetic studies are performed on healthy, euhydrated animals and that the use of NSAIDs in sick neonatal foals may result in altered disposition of drug and adverse effects.

Local anesthetics work through inhibition of sodium channels on nerve fibers preventing impulse propagation to the central nervous system for recognition and interpretation. Aside from regional anesthesia during surgical procedures, lidocaine can be administered IV for analgesia and a reduction in inhalant anesthetic requirements in horses.[36-38] The pharmacokinetics of a lidocaine infusion in anesthetized neonatal horses has not been reported. However, the clinical impression by the authors is that neonatal foals require substantially lower infusion rates than adult horses to achieve inhalant anesthetic reduction. It is important to understand that the pKa (approximately 7.7) of lidocaine is similar to physiologic pH and therefore undergoes ionization in a lower pH. This can result in the phenomenon of ion trapping, whereby the drug enters a compartment and then becomes ionized. As a result, toxic levels of the drug can occur resulting in adverse events. This is of particular concern in pregnant mares near parturition. Lidocaine administration to a mare during anesthesia may result in toxic levels accumulating in the fetus because fetal pH is lower than maternal.[39] Foals delivered from mares with dystocia receiving lidocaine may have systemic levels of lidocaine that interfere with resuscitation efforts.

Induction Agents

The goal of induction of a neonatal foal is rapid unconsciousness and the ability to quickly secure a patent airway. Immobility and muscle relaxation are also necessary to facilitate tracheal intubation, transportation of the foal to a surgical table, and positioning of the foal to allow for appropriate access for a surgical or therapeutic procedure. Induction drugs used in neonatal foals include inhalant anesthetics, ketamine, propofol, and alfaxalone.

Nasotracheal intubation can be performed in awake neonatal foals and then induction of anesthesia can be performed with inhalant anesthetics. This can be particularly useful in depressed, recumbent foals; however, in alert, healthy foals, this method can be stressful and the amount of inhalant anesthetic required to induce anesthesia may result in profound vasodilation and hypotension.

Ketamine, an N-methyl-D-aspartate receptor antagonist, is likely the most commonly used induction agent in horses. Induction with ketamine is typically a stressful event associated with centrally mediated catecholamine release and preservation of cardiovascular parameters.[40] Interestingly, ketamine directly has cardiovascular depressant effects and may result in decreased cardiac function in animals that have little to no catecholamine reserves.[41]

Propofol is a phenolic, nonbarbiturate, short-acting, anesthetic agent that has gained considerable popularity in veterinary medicine owing to rapid induction and termination of effects. It is thought to work through potentiation of gamma-aminobutyric acid receptor activity, the major inhibitory neurotransmitter system in the central nervous system. In horses, propofol is gaining popularity, particularly to improve the quality of recovery; however, there are few published data on its use in foals. Many veterinarians routinely use propofol for induction of foals and the clinical impression is that it provides for a rapid, smooth induction and recovery. Propofol can be used as a sole agent for induction and maintenance of anesthesia in foals and maybe particularly useful for imaging studies.[42] Dose-dependent hypotension is among the more problematic adverse effects of propofol.

Alfaxalone is a neurosteroid similar in structure to progesterone that acts as a nonbarbiturate, short-acting anesthetic agent. Alfaxalone was reintroduced recently into the United Stated and is quickly gaining popularity in equine anesthesia. Alfaxalone has been used for induction and maintenance of anesthesia in ponies and horses.[43,44] The pharmacokinetics and pharmacodynamics of alfaxalone in neonatal foals has been reported.[45] The duration of anesthesia after a single bolus injection of 3 mg/kg was approximately 18 minutes. Oxygen supplementation is recommended because some foals became hypoxemic.

Maintenance Agents

For most veterinary patients, inhalant anesthetics are the mainstay for maintenance of anesthesia, and neonatal foals are no different. Inhalant anesthetics can also be used for induction of anesthesia in neonatal foals.[46] Isoflurane and sevoflurane are the most commonly used anesthetics within the United States. A recent review of inhaled anesthetics in horses was published and the reader is directed there for more detailed information.[47] For the practitioner required to anesthetize a neonatal foal, a working knowledge of the clinical side effects associated with inhalant anesthetics is crucial.

All inhalant anesthetics cause dose dependent cardiovascular depression in adult horses that is defined by vasodilation, and decreased stroke volume and cardiac output.[48–50] Similar changes in foals can be expected. However, the neonatal heart is morphologically immature and is adapted to a low-pressure, hypoxemic environment and the autonomic innervation of the heart may be immature in neonates; therefore, foals may have a limited ability to respond to hypotension and are unable to make proper adjustments in heart rate and vascular resistance.[51] Short- and long-term abnormal neurologic outcomes have been identified in human neonates secondary to hypotension from drug administration.[52]

Horses are extremely sensitive to the dose-dependent respiratory effects of inhalant anesthetics. This manifests clinically as hypoventilation (decreased rate and depth of breathing) with a progression toward apnea as anesthetic dose exceeds one and a half times minimum alveolar concentration.[42,49,50] Neonates have a delicate balance between closing volume and functional residual capacity making them at greater risk to the ventilator complications associated with general anesthesia. Additionally, neonates, whether healthy or diseased, can have an irregular breathing pattern including periodic apnea because of immaturity of the respiratory center in the brain stem. Neonates may also have an altered response to carbon dioxide as a drive for ventilation.[53] Inhalant anesthetic can further disrupt the drive and control of ventilation making severe hypoventilation and need for support during anesthesia highly likely. Lung-protecting strategies such as avoiding excessively high tidal volumes, excessively high airway pressures, use of recruitment maneuvers as needed, and appropriate positive end-expiratory pressure may be beneficial.[53]

PREPARATION FOR ANESTHESIA

Preparation is often key to a successful anesthetic event. Having a preanesthetic checklist to ensure necessary equipment and supplies are available along with a list of concerns for each individual patient can be beneficial in this regard. The equipment required may vary depending on the reason for anesthesia, but should minimally include a source of oxygen and intubation supplies, including multiple sizes of endotracheal tubes to secure the airway. Overnight fasting is recommended for adult horses before anesthesia; however, neonates with their inadequate glycogen stores can be allowed to nurse until the time of anesthesia to prevent hypoglycemia and dehydration. In the healthy foal undergoing an elective procedure, a minimum laboratory database should include packed cell volume, total solids, and a blood glucose; sick neonates may require more extensive biochemical tests indicated earlier to evaluate acid–base, electrolyte, and vital organ function.

Premedication

Premedication before induction of anesthesia is used to decrease stress, provide analgesia, reduce requirements of induction and maintenance drugs, and make the patient more receptive to handling. Obtunded or otherwise compromised patients may not require any premedication. Because of immature organ systems, drug effects may be prolonged; thus, the use of titratable and reversible drugs at doses that produce the desired level of sedation is recommended. The combination of an opioid and a benzodiazepine can often successfully be used in this manner for the neonatal foal. Midazolam or diazepam administered at 0.04 to 0.15 mg/kg along with butorphanol (0.02–0.05 mg/kg) or morphine (0.1 mg/kg) IV often produces a relaxed state allowing for jugular catheter placement and induction of anesthesia. Although older foals may tolerate the cardiovascular depressant effects of alpha-2 agonists, their use in equine neonates is best avoided because decreases in heart rate can decrease cardiac output dramatically and have been associated with greater hemodynamic instability under anesthesia.[4,54] The anesthetist should be aware that neonates are more sensitive to the effects of anesthesia and as a result may respond differently to anesthetic drugs than adults. Careful monitoring of the cardiovascular and pulmonary systems should occur to allow early supportive intervention if necessary.

Induction

Removal of the foal from its dam can be stressful; therefore, dams should be brought to the induction area with their foals to maintain a relaxed environment. Sedation of the dam after validating health may include detomidine (0.005–0.040 mg/kg) or xylazine (0.5–1.0 mg/kg) combined with acepromazine (0.02–0.03 mg/kg) IV. The addition of butorphanol (0.02–0.04 mg/kg) may improve the level of sedation. Once the foal is induced, the mare can be returned to her stall.

After preoxygenation, induction can often be achieved with a combination of ketamine (2.2 mg/kg) and midazolam or diazepam (0.1–0.2 mg/kg) IV, propofol (3–6 mg/kg) IV titrated to effect, or alfaxalone (3 mg/kg) IV titrated to effect. Premedication, disease state, and individual variability can affect dose requirements significantly. Propofol and alfaxalone should be administered slowly because the onset of apnea is dose and rate dependent.[55] Foals may be able to be intubated nasotracheally and induced using inhalant anesthetic, but this method may promote further the development of hypotension and inflict undue stress on the foal.

Intubation

A secure airway gives the anesthetist the ability to deliver inhaled anesthetics and oxygen while decreasing risk of hypoventilation from upper airway obstruction. Intubation in foals is performed blindly, similar to adults, and should be performed with an appropriately sized, lubricated, cuffed endotracheal tube placed either orotracheally (11–16 mm ID) or nasotracheally (7–10 mm ID; **Fig. 1**).

Maintenance

Maintenance of anesthesia can be performed with either injectable anesthetic drugs or, more commonly, with inhaled volatile anesthetic agents. Regardless of method, it is recommended that supplemental oxygen and airway support be available. Both isoflurane and sevoflurane are suitable volatile anesthetics for anesthetizing neonates, but cause dose-dependent cardiovascular and respiratory depression that can be detrimental to the foal. Requirements for maintenance of anesthesia can vary extensively depending on presence of disease, other central nervous system depressant drugs, and hypothermia oftentimes with critically ill neonates requiring minimal if any anesthetic to maintain unconsciousness. The minimum alveolar concentration of isoflurane is demonstrated to be lower in neonatal foals than adults (0.84% vs 1.3%–1.6%) and, when combined with their high minute ventilation, necessitates careful monitoring to avoid anesthetic overdose.[56]

Maintenance of anesthesia using volatile anesthetic agents requires the use of an anesthetic machine. Foals less than 330 lbs (150 kg) can often be accommodated using a small animal anesthetic machine with a precision vaporizer (**Fig. 2**).

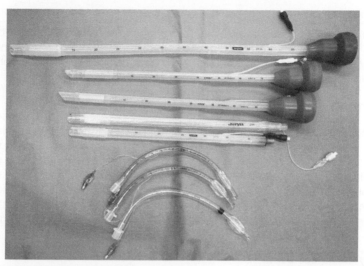

Fig. 1. A variety of endotracheal tube sizes suitable for orotracheal or nasotracheal intubation in the neonatal foal.

For total IV anesthesia, propofol has become popular, being used as either small boluses (1–4 mg/kg) or as a constant rate infusion at 0.2 to 0.4 mg/kg/min to maintain unconsciousness in neonatal foals.[7,42] Likewise, the neurosteroid, alfaxalone, has been investigated for maintenance of anesthesia in adult horses at bolus doses of 0.2 mg/kg or as a constant rate infusion at 3.0 ± 0.6 mg/kg/h.[43] The combination of xylazine (0.5 mg/mL) and ketamine (1–2 mg/mL), in a 5% guaifenesin solution commonly referred to as "triple drip" has been used to maintain anesthesia in older foals, but should be used with caution in neonates owing to unpredictable hemodynamic effects.

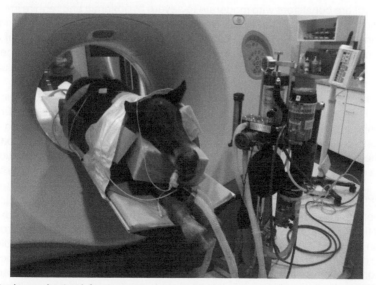

Fig. 2. Foal anesthetized for computed tomography scan using a small animal anesthesia machine with a precision vaporizer.

Positioning

Foals should be positioned on a well-padded surface to prevent uneven distribution of pressure. Inadequate padding is associated with the development of postanesthetic myopathy, and can occur in patients who have prolonged hypotension under anesthesia.[57]

ANESTHETIC MONITORS AND MONITORING

Monitoring vital organ function is a critical part of performing anesthesia in the neonate. Anesthetic monitoring equipment allows complications to be detected early to initiate rapid treatment; however, the benefit of direct interaction with the foal should not be overlooked. Assessment of anesthetic depth, pulse rate and quality, mucous membrane color, capillary refill time, and auscultation of the heart and lungs can provide subjective information concerning circulation, oxygenation, and ventilation and should be performed at regular intervals throughout the anesthetic period.

Assessing Anesthetic Depth

Anesthetic depth as determined by eye position, ocular reflexes, presence of nystagmus, and muscle or anal tone helps the anesthetist avoid too light or too deep a plane of anesthesia. It is important to note, however, that these can sometimes be unreliable in the neonate, and should be interpreted in context of other signs.

Oxygenation and Ventilation

Oxygenation of tissues is often subjectively determined by mucous membrane color and capillary refill time; however, cyanosis is a late sign of hypoxemia (Pao_2 <80 mm Hg) and should not be relied on as a sole indicator of desaturation. Pulse oximetry noninvasively measures the percentage of arterial hemoglobin saturated with oxygen and should be maintained above 95%. Saturations below 90% (Pao_2 <60 mm Hg) are consistent with moderate to severe hypoxemia and require immediate intervention. This monitor additionally allows the anesthetist to assess heart rate and rhythm and in combination with end-tidal CO_2 monitoring is the standard of care in human anesthesia. In sick neonates, cold extremities and poor peripheral perfusion can lead to pulse oximeter error; therefore, in these cases, it is best to evaluate the partial pressure of oxygen (Pao_2) via arterial blood gas analysis.

Subjectively, alveolar ventilation is monitored via observation of respiratory frequency, pulmonary auscultation, and the extent of thoracic excursions. End-tidal CO_2 monitoring via capnometry or capnography is a more accurate way to assess ventilation. End-tidal CO_2 can also be used to confirm endotracheal intubation as well as help to detect low cardiac output states because decreases in end-tidal CO_2 without a change in ventilation can signify a decrease in blood returning to the lungs.[58]

Circulation and Arterial Blood Pressure

Circulation can be assessed via palpation of pulses, auscultation of the thorax, capillary refill time, mucous membrane color, and arterial blood pressure. An electrocardiogram can be used to monitor heart rate and rhythm however, it is not suitable alone because pulseless electrical activity can be present after cardiac arrest has occurred.

Monitoring of arterial blood pressure is advocated as standard of care for anesthetized patients; however, its value in the neonate is controversial because it is notably lower than that of an adult at birth and may take days to months before reaching values considered normal.[59,60] Methods for arterial blood pressure measurement include use of indirect oscillometric devices or Doppler, or direct measurement using an arterial catheter connected to a transducer or aneroid manometer. For longer, more invasive procedures, it is suggested that direct measurement be used whenever possible because indirect methods may be less reliable in the face of severe hypotension. Locations for arterial catheter placement in the foal include the transverse facial, the metatarsal, or the lingual facial arteries.

Although we strive to avoid hypotension, determining what constitutes hypotension in the neonate is difficult. In human neonates, researchers were able to correlate decreases of mean arterial pressure of greater than 15% from awake values with unacceptable levels of cerebral desaturation.[60] This could indicate that mean arterial pressures in the high 40s or 50s may be acceptable, although many still advocate that a minimum of 60 mm Hg be maintained to ensure adequate tissue perfusion.[61] Lacking published data specific to foals, it is recommended that the anesthetist determine acceptable blood pressures as they relate to other measures of tissue perfusion such as blood lactate concentration, heart rate, urine output, and acid–base status.

Temperature

Monitoring body temperature of neonates is of particular importance because hypothermia is a common yet underappreciated complication of anesthesia. Vasodilation of peripheral vessels from anesthetic administration produces a temperature gradient promoting rapid loss of core body heat. This loss is compounded in the neonate owing to a large body surface area to mass ratio, minimal fat stores, depressed thermoregulatory centers in the brain, and poor vasomotor tone. Adverse effects of hypothermia include decreased anesthetic requirements, prolonged recovery, bradycardia, and hypotension unresponsive to catecholamine administration. Methods to prevent and treat hypothermia should be instituted immediately at or before the onset of anesthesia in foals. In dogs and cats, the use of forced air warmers is shown to be superior to other passive methods, such as blankets, for preventing and treating hypothermia.[62] Their use in foals is, therefore, recommended during the perianesthetic period.

Advanced Monitoring Techniques

In certain situations, advanced monitoring of the anesthetized neonate is indicated. Central venous pressure monitoring may be of use in foals where large fluid fluctuations are expected to occur. It can be used as a subjective measure of blood volume. Trends, versus actual numbers, may offer insight regarding response to fluid therapy and identification of fluid overload.[63] Cardiac output monitoring, often restricted to research settings owing to the requirement of a pulmonary arterial catheter or lithium, is now more accessible to the clinician via ultrasound dilution technology only requiring placement of peripheral venous and arterial catheters.[3] The ability to directly identify changes in cardiac output allows the anesthetist to observe the effects of targeted therapies potentially improving anesthetic management.

ADJUNCT ANESTHETIC AND ANALGESIC TECHNIQUES

The dose-dependent cardiovascular and pulmonary depression from volatile anesthetics often results in adverse hypotension, bradycardia, and blunting of protective physiologic reflexes. Balanced anesthesia and analgesia, using lesser doses of multiple drugs to minimize adverse effects from higher individual doses, can often lower the requirement for volatile anesthetics and potentially produce a more stable patient. Ketamine, lidocaine, and several opioids have been investigated for their minimum alveolar concentration–sparing and analgesic effects in the horse, however information in neonates is sparse. Doses in **Table 1** are based on those administered to adult equine patients and although these drugs may offer benefit to the anesthetized foal, caution is warranted when extrapolating doses for the neonate. The immature metabolic capacity of the liver, and changes in liver blood flow and volume of distribution while under anesthesia could lead to higher than expected plasma concentrations and should be taken into consideration when selecting adjunctive drugs.[64]

The benefits of locoregional techniques for decreasing anesthetic requirements should not be overlooked. Peripheral nerve blocks using local anesthetics for lower limb or oral surgeries can provide additional analgesia and prevent transmission of nociceptive information to the spinal cord. Epidural administration of preservative-free morphine (0.1 mg/kg) with saline (0.2 mL/kg total volume) may benefit foals undergoing hind limb or lower abdominal surgeries. Contraindications to epidurals, including sepsis, local infection, and central nervous system disease, should be considered.

COMMON COMPLICATIONS AND THEIR TREATMENT
Hypothermia (See Temperature)

Hypoventilation
Neonates are highly susceptible to the respiratory depressant effects of inhalants and other anesthetic drugs and often require mechanical or assisted ventilation to prevent hypercapnia. Normal partial pressure of carbon dioxide in arterial blood ($Paco_2$) is between 35 and 45 mm Hg with increases above 60 mm Hg associated with the development of hypoxemia when breathing room air, and respiratory acidosis. General guidelines for setting up a mechanical ventilator for the healthy foal include setting the starting tidal volume between 10 and 12 mL/kg with a respiratory frequency of 8 to 12 bpm. The highly compliant thorax of neonatal foals often does not require high peak inspiratory pressures to accommodate this volume and caution should be exercised to avoid volutrauma or barotrauma.

Hypotension
Causes of hypotension under anesthesia include relative (vasodilation) and absolute hypovolemia, bradycardia, and decreased myocardial contractility. In the neonate, cardiac output is heavily dependent on heart rate. The use of anticholinergics to treat hypotension in horses has historically been avoided owing to their effects on gastrointestinal

Table 1			
Adjunct analgesic drugs and doses			
Adjunct Anesthesia/ Analgesia	**Dose**	**Route of Administration**	**Comments**
Fentanyl	0.10–0.30 µg/kg/min	IV	Conflicting evidence regarding MAC reduction
Butorphanol	0.013–0.030 mg/kg/h	IV	—
Ketamine	0.04–0.05 mg/kg/min	IV	—
Lidocaine	35–70 µg/kg/min	IV	Possibility of toxicity owing to decreased metabolic activity

Doses listed are from adults. Caution when extrapolating doses for neonates owing to altered pharmacokinetics and pharmacodynamics
Abbreviations: IV, intravenous; MAC, minimum alveolar concentration.

motility and is often unnecessary in the adult. However, in the presence of bradyarrhythmias that are impacting hemodynamic stability, their judicious use may be justified in the neonatal foal. Foals are susceptible to rapidly developing hypovolemia and may see exaggerated effects owing to an immature baroreceptor reflex.[65] Fluid therapy with crystalloids and/or colloids during anesthesia should be instituted to prevent and treat hypovolemia. Isotonic crystalloids administered at surgical rates of 10 mL/kg/h are often tolerated by healthy foals; however, sick neonates or those undergoing major surgery may have increased fluid requirements or require colloids, such as hetastarch (3–5 mL/kg bolus) to maintain perfusion. A large central compartment, altered hormonal responses, and immature kidneys may also increase risk of fluid overload in the neonate.[65] For this reason, delivery of fluids using a fluid pump may help to avoid accidental excessive fluid administration. Likewise, careful monitoring for serous nasal discharge, nasal edema, chemosis, and pulmonary crackles should be performed.

Inotropes and vasopressors have been examined for treating hypotension in neonatal foals (**Table 2**).[61] Calcium is an inotrope and, when released from the sarcoplasmic reticulum, helps to sustain myocardial contractility. In the face of hypotension, identification and treatment of hypocalcemia may, therefore, improve arterial blood pressure. The short-acting beta agonist, dobutamine, is superior to dopamine for increasing myocardial contractility and arterial blood pressure in foals; however, its effects in very young neonates may be limited by maturity of the heart. The use of vasopressors is often unnecessary in the healthy anesthetized neonate. Septicemia and endotoxemia, however, can produce vasodilatory shock where fluid therapy and inotropes alone are ineffective. Norepinephrine and vasopressin have been investigated in the foal in this regard and may preserve splanchnic perfusion to a greater extent than phenylephrine.[66]

SPECIFIC CONDITIONS OF THE NEONATE
Ruptured Bladder and Uroperiotoneum

Ruptured bladder in the foal can occur from trauma during birth, overexertion, or sequela to local or systemic infection. Electrolyte abnormalities from uroperitoneum

Table 2 Commonly used inotropes and vasopressors in horses		
Agent	**Dose**	**Comments**
Dobutamine	1–5 µg/kg/min	Acts primarily on β1 receptors to improve myocardial contractility. Can be used in conjunction with vasopressor to improve splanchnic blood flow.
10% Calcium gluconate	10–50 mg/kg (0.1–0.5 mL/kg) given over 20–30 min	Can improve myocardial contractility in hypocalcemic patients
Phenylephrine	Load: 2.0 µg/kg bolus CRI: 1.0–3.0 µg/kg/min	Noncatecholamine alpha-1 agonist. Causes significant increase in SVR with decrease in CO.
Norepinephrine	0.05–1.5 µg/kg/min	Primarily alpha-1 agonist with some β1 activity. Often combined with dobutamine to improve MAP and end-organ perfusion.
Vasopressin	0.1–0.5 µU/kg/min	Acts on V2 receptors in vascular smooth muscle to cause vasoconstriction. Works in face of acidemia.

Abbreviations: CO, cardiac output; CRI, constant rate infusion; IV, intravenous; MAP, mean arterial pressure; SVR, systemic vascular resistance.

include hyponatremia, hypochloridemia, hypocalcemia, and potentially life-threatening hyperkalemia, and should be considered a medical emergency requiring stabilization before anesthesia and surgical correction. Addressing fluid deficits and acid–base abnormalities with crystalloids and/or colloids can help to correct electrolyte imbalances.[67] If hyperkalemia is present, 0.9% saline is often used to rapidly lower potassium concentration; however, lactated Ringer solution ($[K^+]$ = 4 mEq/L) is also acceptable. Hyperkalemia is associated with the development of classic changes in the electrocardiogram (tented t waves, flattened p waves, and widening QRS complexes) and the formation of arrhythmias.[68] Patients with a potassium concentration of greater than 5.5 mEq/L (6.0 mEq/L in emergencies) require correction before anesthesia. Slow administration of 10% calcium gluconate (0.3–0.5 mL/kg) will transiently help to balance cell membrane potential while corrective measures are implemented. Dextrose as a 50% solution (1 mL/kg) can be administered with or without the addition of insulin (0.1–0.3 IU/kg) to move potassium into cells. Caution and frequent blood glucose monitoring is advised when administering insulin because hypoglycemia could develop.[68] Once anesthetized, copious fluid administration and manual or mechanical ventilation should be maintained to prevent acid–base derangements that may increase potassium.

Septicemia

Anesthesia of the septic neonate can be challenging no matter the skill set of the anesthetist. The release of cytokines and inflammatory mediators that mark the pathophysiology of sepsis result in vascular endothelial damage and vasodilation, producing hypotension and hypovolemia that are minimally responsive to crystalloid or colloid therapy. Hypoperfusion leads to lactic acidosis and end-organ hypoxia. In septic neonates, stabilization efforts should continue into the anesthetic period because rapidly deteriorating status may necessitate immediate surgery. Placement of additional IV catheters allows rapid administration of fluids or blood products to correct hypovolemia. Serial electrolyte and lactate measurements along with changes in heart rate, blood pressure, urine output, and capillary refill time can help to gauge the success of fluid resuscitation. An infusion of dobutamine (1–5 μg/kg/min) is often necessary to improve myocardial contractility. If this alone does not improve perfusion parameters, the addition of a vasopressor, such as norepinephrine (0.05–1.5 μg/kg/min) or vasopressin (0.1–0.5 μU/kg/min) has been advocated.[61,66] This combination was demonstrated to preserve splanchnic perfusion better than the use of a vasopressor alone.[61] Vasopressin has gained considerable popularity for the treatment of blood pressure in vasodilatory shock because, unlike catecholamines, it continues to work in the face of significant acidemia.[69] Glucose should also be monitored at regular intervals because both hypoglycemia and hyperglycemia are known to occur in sepsis and the administration of dextrose as a 2.5% to 5% solution may be necessary.

Pulmonary Disease

It is not unusual for neonatal foals requiring emergent anesthesia to have coexisting respiratory disease. Hypoxemia from ventilation and perfusion (V/Q) mismatch is of significant concern for this population because anesthesia alone can result in altered matching through atelectasis and changes in gas distribution. Careful attention to pre-oxygenation and monitoring oxygen saturation (SaO_2) and Pao_2 via serial blood gas measurements is necessary. Initiation of mechanical ventilation can help to improve gas exchange in these foals as well as decrease their work of breathing under anesthesia. Other treatments for hypoxemia reported in horses include endotracheal administration of the beta-2 agonist, albuterol via metered dose inhaler, and the use of positive end-expiratory pressure after a recruitment maneuver to help open collapsed alveoli.[70,71] Research using these methods has not been carried out in neonatal foals and the anesthetist is cautioned regarding the risks of volutrauma and barotrauma in this population. Foals with evidence of acute respiratory distress syndrome may actually require lower tidal volumes (6–8 mL/kg) and higher respiratory frequencies to avoid exacerbation of their respiratory compromise.[72] Oxygen supplementation should be continued after recovery along with appropriate monitoring. In foals who cannot maintain a Pao_2 of greater than 60 mm Hg despite oxygen administration, ventilatory support may become necessary.

RECOVERY

After the cessation of anesthesia, foals should be moved to a quiet, warm, and preferably padded recovery stall. Monitoring and oxygen supplementation should be continued throughout the recovery period. Sick foals may additionally require continued administration of vasoactive drugs and fluids. Active warming and drying of the haircoat during recovery can prevent the onset of shivering and is recommended because shivering significantly increases metabolic oxygen demand.[62] Foals with respiratory disease may benefit from being placed in sternal recumbency because this may improve gas exchange. Although foals may or may not demonstrate acute signs of pain, the anesthetist should use behavior and response to gentle wound palpation to help to guide appropriate administration of analgesics. Neonates should be assisted to stand to prevent rough or uncoordinated recoveries. Once stable, the mare can be brought to the recovery area and the pair can be returned to their stall.

SUMMARY

Anesthesia of the equine neonate presents significant challenges to even the most experienced anesthetist. Specific research pertaining to neonatal foal anesthesia is limited and extrapolation from adult literature can be inappropriate in some situations. Despite this limitation, knowledge of neonate physiology, careful preparation, appropriate drug selection, and diligent monitoring can increase chances of a successful outcome.

REFERENCES

1. Johnston GM, Eastment JK, Wood JL, et al. The confidential enquiry into perioperative equine fatalities (CEPEF): mortality results of phases 1 and 2. Vet Anaesth Analg 2002;29(4):159–70.
2. Thomas J. Reducing the risk in neonatal anesthesia. Ped Ananesthesia 2014;24: 106–13.
3. Shih AC, Queiroz P, Vigani A, et al. Comparison of cardiac output determined by an ultrasound velocity dilution cardiac output method and by the lithium dilution cardiac output method in juvenile horses with experimentally induced hypotension. Am J Vet Res 2014;75(6):565–71.
4. Grubb TL, Perez Jimenez TE, Pettifer GR. Anesthesia and analgesia for selected patients or procedures: neonatal and pediatric patients. In: Grimm KA, Lamont LA, Tranquilli WJ, et al, editors. Lumb and Jones veterinary anesthesia and analgesia. 5th edition. Ames (IA): Wiley-Blackwell; 2015. p. 983–7.
5. Dunlop CL. Anesthesia and sedation in foals. Vet Clin North Am Equine Pract 1994;10:67–85.

6. Schliewert EC, Lascola KM, O'Brien RT, et al. Comparison of radiographic and computed tomographic images of the lungs in healthy neonatal foals. Am J Vet Res 2015;76(1):42–52.

7. Lascola KM, O'Brien RT, Wilkins PA, et al. Qualitative and quantitative interpretation of computed tomography of the lungs in healthy neonatal foals. Am J Vet Res 2013;74(9):1239–46.

8. McNally EM, Robertson SA, Pablo LS. Comparison of time to desaturation between preoxygenated and nonpreoxygenated dogs following sedation with acepromazine maleate and morphine and induction of anesthesia with propofol. Am J Vet Res 2009;70(11):1333–8.

9. Carter SW, Roberstoan SA, Steel CJ, et al. Cardiopulmonary effects of xylazine sedation in the foal. Equine Vet J 1990;22(6):384–8.

10. Rutkowski JA, Ross MW, Cullen K. Effects of xylazine and/or butorphanol or neostigmine on myoelectric activity of the cecum and right ventral colon in female ponies. Am J Vet Res 1989;50(7):1096–101.

11. Rutkowski JA, Eades SC, Moore JN. Effects of xylazine butorphanol on cecal arterial blood flow, cecal mechanical activity, and systemic hemodynamics in horses. Am J Vet Res 1991;52(7):1153–8.

12. Eades SC, Moore JN. Blockade of endotoxin-induced cecal hypoperfusion and ileus with an alpha 2 antagonist in horses. Am J Vet Res 1993;54(4):586–90.

13. Nuñez E, Steffey EP, Ocampo L, et al. Effects of alpha2-adrenergic receptor agonists on urine production in horses deprived of food and water. Am J Vet Res 2004;65(10):1342–6.

14. Lim TY, Poole RL, Pageler NM. Propylene glycol toxicity in children. J Pediatr Pharmacol Ther 2014;19(4):277–82.

15. Hubbell JA, Kelly EM, Aarnes TL, et al. Pharmacokinetics of midazolam after intravenous administration to horses. Equine Vet J 2013;45(6):721–5.

16. Massoco C, Palermo-Neto J. Effects of midazolam on equine innate immune response: a flow cytometric study. Vet Immunol Immunopathol 2003;95(1–2): 11–9.

17. Pequito M, Amory H, de Moffarts B, et al. Evaluation of acepromazine-induced hemodynamic alterations and reversal with norepinephrine infusion in standing horses. Can Vet J 2013;54(2):150–6.

18. Anand KJ, Sippell WG, Aynsley-Green A. Randomised trial of fentanyl anaesthesia in preterm babies undergoing surgery: effects on the stress response. Lancet 1987;1:243–8.

19. Anand KJ, Hickey PR. Haltohane-morphine compared with high-dose sufentanil for anesthesia and postoperative analgesia in neonatal cardiac surgery. N Engl J Med 1992;326:1–9.

20. Bromage PR, Shibata HR, Willoughby HW. Influence of prolonged epidural blockade on blood sugar and cortisol responses to operations upon the upper part of the abdomen and the thorax. Surg Gynecol Obstet 1971;132: 1051–6.

21. Goldman RD, Koren G. Biologic markers of pain in the vulnerable infant. Clin Perinatol 2002;29:415–25.

22. Knych HK, Steffey EP, Mama KR, et al. Effects of high plasma fentanyl concentrations on minimum alveolar concentration of isoflurane in horses. Am J Vet Res 2009;70(10):1193–200.

23. Knych HK, Steffey EP, McKemie DS. Preliminary pharmacokinetics of morphine and its major metabolites following intravenous administration of four doses to horses. J Vet Pharmacol Ther 2014;37(4):374–81.

24. Knych HK, Steffey EP, Casbeer HC, et al. Disposition, behavioural and physiological effects of escalating doses of intravenously administered fentanyl to young foals. Equine Vet J 2015;47(5):592–8.
25. Knych HK, Steffey EP, Mitchell MM, et al. Effects of age on the pharmacokinetics and selected pharmacodynamics of intravenously administered fentanyl in foals. Equine Vet J 2015;47(1):72–7.
26. Love EJ, Taylor PM, Murrell J, et al. Effects of acepromazine, butorphanol and buprenorphine on thermal and mechanical nociceptive thresholds in horses. Equine Vet J 2012;44:221–5.
27. Sanchez LC, Robertson SA. Pain control in horses: what do we really know? Equine Vet J 2014;46:517–23.
28. Arquedas MG, Hines MT, Papich MG, et al. Pharmacokinetics of butorphanol and evaluation of physiologic and behavioral effects after intravenous and intramuscular administration to neonatal foals. J Vet Intern Med 2008;22(6):1417–26.
29. McGowan KT, Elfenbein JR, Roberston SA, et al. Effects of butorphanol on thermal nociceptive threshold in healthy pony foals. Equine Vet J 2013;45(4): 503–6.
30. Santos LC, de Moraes AN, Saito ME. Effects of intraarticular ropivacaine and morphine on lipopolysaccharide-induced synovitis in horses. Vet Anaesth Analg 2009;36(3):280–6.
31. van Loon JP, de Grauw JC, van Dierendonck M, et al. Intra-articular opioid analgesia is effective in reducing pain and inflammation in an equine LPS induced synovitis model. Equine Vet J 2010;42(5):412–9.
32. Wilcke JR, Crisman MV, Sams RA, et al. Pharmacokinetics of phenylbutazone in neonatal foals. Am J Vet Res 1993;54(12):2064 7.
33. Semrad SD, Sams RA, Ashcraft SM. Pharmacokinetics of and serum thromboxane suppression by flunixin meglumine in healthy foals during the first month of life. Am J Vet Res 1993;54(12):2083–7.
34. Raidal SL, Edwards S, Pippia J, et al. Pharmacokinetics and safety of oral administration of meloxicam to foals. J Vet Intern Med 2013;27(2):300–7.
35. Hovanessian N, Davis JL, McKenzie HC 3rd, et al. Pharmacokinetics and safety of firocoxib after oral administration of repeated consecutive doses to neonatal foals. J Vet Pharmacol Ther 2014;37(3):243–51.
36. Wagner AE, Mama KR, Steffey EP, et al. Comparison of the cardiovascular effects of equipotent anesthetic doses of sevoflurane alone and sevoflurane plus an intravenous infusion of lidocaine in horses. Am J Vet Res 2011;72(4):452–60.
37. Rezende ML, Wagner AE, Mama KR, et al. Effects of intravenous administration of lidocaine on the minimum alveolar concentration of sevoflurane in horses. Am J Vet Res 2011;72(4):446–51.
38. Robertson SA, Sanchez LC, Merritt AM, et al. Effect of systemic lidocaine on visceral and somatic nociception in conscious horses. Equine Vet J 2005;37(2): 122–7.
39. Biehl D, Shnider SM, Levinson G, et al. Placental transfer of lidocaine: effects of fetal acidosis. Anesthesiology 1978;48(6):409–12.
40. Carruba MO, Bondiolotti G, Picotti GB, et al. Effects of diethyl ether, halothane, ketamine and urethane on sympathetic activity in the rat. Eur J Pharmacol 1987;134(1):15–24.
41. Zausig YA, Busse H, Lunz D, et al. Cardiac effects of induction agents in the septic rat heart. Crit Care 2009;13(5):R144.
42. Chaffin MK, Walker MA, McArthur NH, et al. Magnetic resonance imaging of the brain of normal neonatal foals. Vet Radiol Ultrasound 1997;38(2):102–11.

43. Klöppel H, Leece EA. Comparison of ketamine and alfaxalone for induction and maintenance of anaesthesia in ponies undergoing castration. Vet Anaesth Analg 2011;38(1):37–43.
44. Keates HL, van Eps AW, Pearson MR. Alfaxalone compared with ketamine for induction of anaesthesia in horses following xylazine and guaifenesin. Vet Anaesth Analg 2012;39(6):591–8.
45. Goodwin W, Keates H, Pasloske K, et al. Plasma pharmacokinetics and pharmacodynamics of alfaxalone in neonatal foals after an intravenous bolus of alfaxalone following premedication with butorphanol tartrate. Vet Anaesth Analg 2012;39(5):503–10.
46. Steffey EP, Willits N, Wong P, et al. Clinical investigations of halothane and isoflurane for induction and maintenance of foal anesthesia. J Vet Pharmacol Ther 1991; 14(3):300–9.
47. Brosnan RJ. Inhaled anesthetics in horses. Vet Clin North Am Equine Pract 2013; 29(1):69–87.
48. Steffey EP, Howland D Jr. Comparison of circulatory and respiratory effects of isoflurane and halothane anesthesia in horses. Am J Vet Res 1980;41(5):821–5.
49. Steffey EP, Mama KR, Faley FD, et al. Effects of sevoflurane dose and mode of ventilation on cardiopulmonary function and blood biochemical variable in horses. Am J Vet Res 2005;66(4):606–14.
50. Steffey EP, Woliner MJ, Puschner B, et al. Effects of desflurane and mode of ventilation on cardiovascular and respiratory functions and clinicopathologic variables in horses. Am J Vet Res 2005;66(4):669–77.
51. Wolf AR, Humphry AT. Limitations and vulnerabilities of the neonatal cardiovascular system: considerations for anesthetic management. Paediatr Anaesth 2014; 24(1):5–9.
52. Anand KJ, Hall RW, Desai N, et al. Effects of morphine analgesia in ventilated preterm neonates: primary outcomes from the NEOPAIN randomized trial. Lancet 2004;363(9422):1673–82.
53. Neumann RP, von Ungem-Sternberg BS. The neonatal lung—physiology and ventilation. Paediatr Anaesth 2014;24(1):10–21.
54. Kerr CL, Boure LP, Pearce SG, et al. Cardiopulmonary effects of diazepam-ketamine-isoflurane or xylazine-ketamine-isoflurane during abdominal surgery in foals. Am J Vet Res 2009;70:574–80.
55. Amengual M, Flaherty D, Auckburally A, et al. An evaluation of anaesthetic induction in healthy dogs using rapid intravenous injection of propofol or alfaxalone. Vet Anaesth Analg 2013;40:115–23.
56. Dunlop CS, Hodgson DS, Grandy JL, et al. The MAC of isoflurane in foals. Vet Surg 1989;18:247–54.
57. Manning M, Dubielzig R, McGuirk S. Postoperative myositis in a neonatal foal: a case report. Vet Surg 1995;24:69–72.
58. Kodali BS, Urman RD. Capnography during cardiopulmonary resuscitation: current evidence and future directions. J Emerg Trauma Shock 2014;7(4): 332–40.
59. Magrini F. Haemodynamic determinants of the arterial blood pressure rise during growth in conscious puppies. Cardiovasc Res 1978;12(7):422–8.
60. Michelet D, Arslan O, Hilly J, et al. Intraoperative changes in blood pressure associated with cerebral desaturation in infants. Pediatric Anesthesia 2015;25: 681–8.
61. Corley KTT. Inotropes and vasopressors in adults and foals. Vet Clin Equine 2004; 20:77–106.

62. Clark-Price S. Inadvertent perianesthetic hypothermia in small animal patients. Vet Clin North Am Small Anim Pract 2015;45(5):983–94. Available at: http://dx. doi.org/10.1016/j.cvsm.2015.04.005.
63. Haskins SC. Monitoring anesthestized patients. In: Grimm KA, Lamont LA, Tranquilli WJ, et al, editors. Lumb and Jones veterinary anesthesia and analgesia. 5th edition. Ames (IA): Wiley-Blackwell; 2015. p. 86–113.
64. Gozalo-Marcilla M, Gasthuys F, Schauvliege S. Partial intravenous anaesthesia in the horse: a review of intravenous agents used to supplement equine inhalation anaesthesia. Part 1: lidocaine and ketamine. Vet Anaesth Analg 2014;41:335–45.
65. Hollis AR, Boston RC. Corley KTT Plasma aldosterone, vasopressin and atrial natriuretic peptide in hypovolaemia: a preliminary comparative study of neonatal and mature horses. Equine Vet J 2008;40(1):64–9.
66. Dickey EJ, McKenzie HC, Johnson A, et al. Use of pressor therapy in 34 hypotensive critically ill neonatal foals. Aust Vet J 2010;88:472–7.
67. Dunkel B, Palmer JE, Olson KN, et al. Uroperitoneum in 32 foals: influence of intravenous fluid therapy, infection, and sepsis. J Vet Intern Med 2005;19(6): 889–93.
68. Dibartola SP, de Morais HA. Disorders of potassium: hypokalemia and hyperkalemia. In: Dibartola SP, editor. Fluid, electrolyte, and acid-base disorders in small animal practice. 3rd edition. St. Louis: Saunders Elsevier; 2006. p. 91–121.
69. Kawano T, Tanaka K, Nazari H, et al. The effects of extracellular pH on vasopressin inhibition of ATP-sensitive K+ channels in vascular smooth muscle cells. Anesth Analg 2007;105:1714–9.
70. Robertson SA, Bailey JE. Aerosolized salbutamol (albuterol) improves PaO2 in hypoxaemic anaesthetized horses—a prospective clinical trial in 81 horses. Vet Anaesth Analg 2002;29:212–8.
71. Hopster K, Kastner S, Rohn K, et al. Intermittent positive pressure ventilation with constant positive end-expiratory pressure and alveolar recruitment manoeuvre during inhalation anaesthesia in horses undergoing surgery for colic, and its influence on the early recovery period. Vet Anaesth Analg 2011;38:169–77.
72. Palmer JE. Ventilatory support of the critically ill foal. Vet Clin Equine 2005;21: 457–86.

The Equine Neonatal Central Nervous System
Development and Diseases

Brett S. Tennent-Brown, BSc, DipSc, BVSc, MS[a],*,
Ashleigh V. Morrice, BSc, DVM[a], Stephen Reed, DVM[b]

KEYWORDS

- Neonatal encephalopathy • Neurosteroids • Allopregnanolone • Progestagens

KEY POINTS

- Neonatal encephalopathy (neonatal maladjustment syndrome, hypoxic-ischemic enceph-alopathy) is the most common neurologic condition affecting newborn foals and shares similarities with perinatal asphyxia syndrome of human infants.
- In many cases of neonatal encephalopathy there is no obvious episode of acute or chronic hypoxia and other mechanisms likely play a role in the pathogenesis.
- The role of neurosteroids in neonatal encephalopathy has been investigated and increased concentrations of neuroactive progestagens are found in affected foals; whe-ther these molecules are protective, as has been suggested, or play a role in the patho-genesis is unknown.
- Neurologic diseases other than neonatal encephalopathy affect foals occasionally and should be considered when evaluating sick foals with clinical signs of neurologic dysfunction.

INTRODUCTION

Neonatal encephalopathy (NE; neonatal maladjustment syndrome [NMS], hypoxic-ischemic encephalopathy [HIE]) is the most common disease affecting the central nervous system (CNS) of equine neonates. The condition has often been compared with perinatal asphyxia syndrome (PAS) in human infants but it seems likely that oxygen deprivation during gestation or parturition is not the only mechanism by which NE occurs. In a subset of foals, NE might occur as a result of an inflammatory insult or from

Funding Sources: None.
Conflicts of Interest: None.
[a] Equine Centre, Faculty of Veterinary and Agricultural Sciences, The University of Melbourne, 250 Princess Highway, Werribee, Victoria 3030, Australia; [b] Rood and Riddle Equine hospital, 2150 Georgetown Road, Lexington, KY 40511, USA
* Corresponding author.
E-mail address: brett.tennent@unimelb.edu.au

failure to make the transition from intrauterine to extrauterine life. Several recent studies have focused on the role of a group of molecules termed neurosteroids that influence alertness and arousal of the fetus and seem to be important in the onset of consciousness in neonates. The bulk of this article discusses aspects of the endocrine changes that occur at birth and the role that these changes might play in NE. Other conditions affecting the equine neonatal brain are covered only briefly and interested readers are directed to an excellent recent review.[1]

CENTRAL NERVOUS SYSTEM DEVELOPMENT IN THE FETUS
The Hypothalamic-Pituitary-Adrenal Axis and the Transition from Intrauterine to Extrauterine Life

The fetal hypothalamic-pituitary-adrenal (HPA) axis plays a pivotal role in the transition from intrauterine to extrauterine life (recently reviewed by Fowden and colleagues,[2] 2012). Furthermore, the pattern of cortisol and steroid hormone secretion by the fetal adrenal gland is an important signal in initiating labor. Before 290 days of gestation, fetal pituitary secretion of adrenocorticotropic hormone is low and the adrenal glands produce mainly pregnenolone (a steroid hormone precursor synthesized from cholesterol). Fetal pregnenolone is thought to be the main precursor for the progestagens synthesized by the uteroplacental tissues. These progestagens are responsible for maintaining the uterus in a quiescent state if there is increased stretching by the fetus.[3–6] Fetal HPA axis activity increases and is accompanied by adrenal gland development after 300 days of gestation. Very late in gestation, in just the last 24 to 48 hours before parturition, the fetal adrenal switches from pregnenolone production to cortisol production. Fetal pregnenolone concentrations consequently decrease; removal of this precursor results in a sharp decrease in maternal progestagen concentration and an increase in uterine activity. The concomitant increase in fetal cortisol concentration facilitates maturation of a wide range of body systems that are essential to extrauterine life, including the respiratory, gastrointestinal, hepatic, and renal systems.[7,8] Normal HPA axis development and function are disrupted by both prematurity and sepsis, and the degree of disruption seems to have an important influence on the occurrence of disease and survival of affected neonates.[9–12]

Neurosteroids in Central Nervous System Development and Function

The neurosteroids are a collection of steroid hormones synthesized from cholesterol or other circulating steroids by enzymes located within the CNS.[13] These molecules are thought to be important in the transition to extrauterine life and the onset of consciousness[14,15] but also have roles in neurologic function and disease in the fetus, neonate, and adult.[13] As with traditional steroid hormones, the neurosteroids can modulate gene expression; however, they also have important and much more rapid actions at several neurotransmitter receptors, including the gamma-aminobutyric acid (GABA) A and N-methyl-D-aspartate (NMDA) receptors.[13]

GABA is the most important inhibitory neurotransmitter within the mammalian CNS and the $GABA_A$ receptors are a family of ligand-gated anion channels.[16] There are approximately 20 to 30 isoforms of the $GABA_A$ receptor with distinct physiologic properties.[17] Combined with differing regional expression of the $GABA_A$ receptors throughout the CNS, this results in a high degree of specificity.[17] The neurosteroids probably do not function by themselves at the $GABA_A$ receptor but potentiate the action of GABA (and possibly other ligands) at the receptor.[13] Neurosteroid binding at the $GABA_A$ receptor generally has a depressant effect on the CNS as a result of increased GABAergic inhibition and anion (chloride ion) influx.

Because of its precocious nature, the ungulate fetus is neurologically mature and capable of conscious perception at birth but is maintained in a sleeplike state throughout gestation.[18] Inhibition of fetal CNS activity and movement is thought to protect the dam against injury during gestation but might also be protective for the fetus (discussed later). This unconscious state is maintained by both physical and chemical factors, including high concentrations of neuroactive progesterone metabolites.[14,18,19] Progesterone and allopregnanolone are found in high concentrations in the fetal circulation and brain, respectively, and are considered the most important neuroactive steroids present in the fetus during pregnancy.[20] Allopregnanolone, which is synthesized from progesterone by the action of 5α-reductase, seems to be the key neurosteroid responsible for suppressing fetal CNS activity.

Placental progesterone synthesis during late gestation supplies the fetal brain with high concentrations of progesterone for allopregnanolone synthesis. Administration of (additional) progesterone to the dam or administration of pregnanolone directly to the fetus suppresses arousal-like behavior in fetal sheep.[21,22] In contrast, reduction in placental progesterone synthesis following administration of trilostane (a 3β-hydroxysteroid dehydrogenase inhibitor that reduces conversion of pregnenolone to progesterone) decreases sleeplike behavior and increases the incidence of arousal-like activity in fetal sheep. Arousal-like behavior decreases back to control levels when progesterone is administrated after trilostane treatment.[14] Inhibition of 5α-reductase by administration of finasteride to fetal sheep increases fetal behavior suggestive of arousal.[23] At parturition, loss of the progesterone source (ie, the placenta) is suggested to cause a rapid decrease in the concentrations of neuroinhibitory progesterone metabolites, allowing the transition to a postnatal state of consciousness.

In addition to their role in inhibiting CNS activity and movement in the fetus, the neurosteroids seem to have a major role in CNS development and remodeling. Reduction of brain allopregnanolone concentrations by administration of finasteride in late gestation causes widespread apoptosis in the brain of fetal sheep.[24] This apoptosis might have implications for preterm neonates because those neonates are expected to experience a decrease in neurosteroid concentrations earlier in their development. The neurosteroids also seem to be involved in myelination, axonal growth, and dendritic growth, and might act to refine synaptic connections.[25]

The Role of Neurosteroids in Neonatal Neurologic Disease

Circulating and, particularly, cerebral concentrations of allopregnanolone are high in the fetus but increase further during periods of stress and hypoxia.[26] Hypoxia induced in late gestation by brief (10 minutes) occlusion of umbilical blood flow produces a sustained increase in allopregnanolone concentration in both the gray and white matter of the fetal sheep brain.[27] The asphyxia-induced increase in allopregnanolone concentration results from upregulation of expression of the enzymes responsible for synthesizing the neurosteroid. Chronic placental insufficiency causing fetal hypoxemia and in utero growth restriction leads to chronic increases in 5α-reductase expression and allopregnanolone synthesis in the brains of fetal guinea pigs and sheep.[28]

Postnatal stressors can also cause increases in brain neurosteroid concentrations. The effects of hypoxia or administration of lipopolysaccharide (LPS) and a combination of both have been assessed in newborn lambs. Both hypoxia and LPS administration caused marked increases in brain allopregnanolone concentrations and this increase was greater still when hypoxia followed LPS administration.[29,30] Allopregnanolone concentrations were increased in all brain areas except the cerebellum and diencephalon following administration of LPS to neonatal lambs and it was suggested that the LPS-induced increase in allopregnanolone might contribute to the somnolence seen in sick neonates.[30] These studies and others suggest that although allopregnanolone concentrations decrease rapidly after birth in the normal neonate, concentrations in the brain might increase again (or remain increased) in response to a range of postnatal stressors.[29,30]

The Neuroprotective Role of Allopregnanolone and the Other Neurosteroids

It has been suggested that the increase in allopregnanolone concentrations in response to hypoxemia or other stressors might be a protective response rather than a component of the disorder.[28] Considerable evidence supports a neuroprotective role for allopregnanolone in adult models of traumatic and hypoxic-ischemic brain injury.[31,32] Progesterone concentrations influence the frequency and severity of seizure activity in women with epilepsy, and allopregnanolone (derived from progesterone) is thought to have anticonvulsant activity.[13] Neuroprotection is a consequence of GABA$_A$ receptor—mediated hyperpolarization resulting in reduced neuronal excitation with subsequent reduced susceptibility to excitotoxic cell death.[33]

Increases in neurosteroid concentration might also limit brain injury in the fetus. Increased allopregnanolone concentration within the fetal brain is thought to reduce the adverse effects of hypoxia, protecting against further insults and limiting cell death. Infusion of pregnanolone into the fetal circulation reduces CNS excitability and blocks the convulsant actions of GABAergic antagonists in fetal sheep brains.[34] If the increase in cerebral allopregnanolone synthesis is suppressed by administration of the 5α-reductase inhibitor finasteride a significant increase in apoptosis occurs following asphyxia, particularly within the hippocampus.[35] It has been further suggested that the decrease in brain allopregnanolone concentrations in the normal neonate might increase its susceptibility to brain injury.[35,36]

Progestagen Concentrations in Neonatal Foals

Progestagens, progestogens, or progestins refer to a series of progesterone and pregnenolone metabolites present in equine maternal and fetal plasma.[4] Progestagens are either pregnenes (unsaturated steroids) or pregnanes (saturated steroids).[4] A range of progesterone metabolites, primarily the 5α-pregnanes, are produced by the equine placenta but, within the fetus, pregnenolone and its metabolites predominate.[4,5,19] In healthy foals, plasma progestagen concentrations are high at birth and then decrease rapidly over the first day of life, presumably as a result of the loss of placentally derived precursors, so that they are almost undetectable by the second day postpartum.[4,19,37,38] The decrease in plasma concentrations of these hormones, some of which have a neuromodulatory role, is thought to be a component of the transition from intrauterine to extrauterine life and the onset of consciousness.[18] Plasma progestagen concentrations remain high after parturition and can increase further in foals with a range of equine neonatal diseases, including those with a clinical diagnosis of NE.[37–39] Progestagen concentrations are higher in more severely compromised foals, tending to increase as the foal's condition deteriorates and decrease as condition improves.[37–39]

Based on their neuroinhibitory effects, it has been suggested that increased concentrations of neuroactive progestagens contribute to the pathogenesis of equine NE, particularly in those foals in which there is not an obvious episode of asphyxia.[39,40] Supporting this, infusion of allopregnanolone to a healthy, neurologically normal foal resulted in the temporary development of clinical signs similar to those of NE.[40] Increased progestagen concentrations in foals with NE might result from failure of appropriate transition signals caused by rapid passage through the birth canal or caesarian delivery. Alternatively, postpartum events might cause a reversion to a fetal hormonal state. However, as discussed, the increase in progestagen derivatives in sick neonatal foals might represent a protective response to limit brain injury rather than a component of the disease process.[28] Progestagen concentrations, including progestagens that are considered to be active within the CNS, are also increased in foals with conditions other than NE, including sepsis.[37–39] Further, concentrations of neuroactive progestagens are increased in foals that have experienced an episode of hypoxia as well as those in which an obvious hypoxic event was not appreciated.[39]

CLINICAL ASSESSMENT OF THE NEONATAL CENTRAL NERVOUS SYSTEM

A thorough, consistent neurologic examination is essential during the initial evaluation of foals with neurologic disease and when monitoring their progression. A detailed neurologic examination appropriate for equine neonates has been described[1]; however-er, it is worth emphasizing some of the behavioral characteristics that might provide important early insights into the neurologic status of a newborn foal. Normal foals should be sternal within 5 minutes and have a suckle reflex within 20 minutes (although this is often present immediately after birth). Most foals stand within an hour of partu-rition but clinicians might need to allow a little extra time for foals trying to stand on hard, slippery floors or for foals that are very large. Normal foals quickly find the mare's udder and most have nursed by 2 hours of age, although some normal foals can take longer than this. The foal's awareness of its environment should also be carefully eval-uated; although inquisitive about their surroundings, most normal neonates remain very close to their dams. Gastrointestinal function can be disrupted in foals that have experienced a period of hypoxia; healthy foals often defecate soon after standing or following their first meal but some normal foals do not defecate for 24 hours.

The pupils in foals 1 to 2 days old should be equal in size, large, and circular, decreasing in size and becoming more ovoid over the first week of life. Direct and in-direct pupillary light reflexes should be present but the rate of pupillary constriction can be influenced by the degree of excitement. Neonatal foals do not develop a menace response until about 2 weeks of age on average because this is a learned behavior. When the foal's head is manipulated, it is normal to observe an exaggerated physiologic, horizontal nystagmus with the fast phase in the direction of head move-ment. Movements of newborn foals are typically swift and can appear jerky; stimula-tion often results in an exaggerated response that should not be confused with the hyperresponsiveness associated with NE. Normal foals may allow their tongue to hang out of the mouth but are able to completely withdraw it when stimulated. Normal foals also display a crossed extensor reflex that can last for up to 3 weeks and a brisk patellar reflex can be observed in many normal foals.

NEONATAL ENCEPHALOPATHY

The term NE has been used to refer to a noninfectious syndrome of foals primarily characterized by CNS dysfunction. NE has several synonyms, including HIE, NMS, dummy foal syndrome, and wanderer or barker foals. This variety of names reflects the predominant clinical features of some of these cases but also highlight the lack of a complete understanding of the disease. The incidence of NE has been reported at 1% to 2% of all foal births or 0.75% of thoroughbred births[41]; however, lack of both a specific clinical definition and diagnostic tools to make a definitive diagnosis makes precise calculations of incidence difficult.

NE shares some features of PAS in human infants and is often associated with peri-partum events such as dystocia, cesarean section, premature placental separation, or placentitis in which there is a cause of acute or chronic hypoxia. The pathophysiology of HIE has recently been thoroughly reviewed.[42] An early report described necrosis and hemorrhage of the brain in a necropsy study of a small group of severely affected foals.[41] However, there is often no evidence of hypoxic-ischemic or hemorrhagic brain injury or cerebral edema in foals clinically diagnosed with NE and, in many cases, an obvious cause of hypoxia is not apparent. Furthermore, many foals with NE make a complete and rapid recovery in stark contrast to animal models of perinatal asphyxia and affected human infants.[43,44] Human studies report NE occurring after in utero exposure to infection or inflammation and the subsequent cascade of proinflammatory cytokine[45,46] and clinical experience suggests that this might also occur in foals. Proinflammatory cytokines could cause CNS injury via a myriad of pathways, including direct cytotoxicity, increased blood-brain barrier permeability, changes in vascular tone and tissue perfusion, and increased release of excitotoxic neurotransmitters. Recently the role of neuroactive progestagens has been investigated in foals with a clinical diagnosis of NE (and other neonatal diseases).[39] As described earlier, increased concentration of allopregnanolone and, probably, other neurosteroids might be responsible for at least some of the clinical signs of NE. However, whether the increase in the neuroactive progestagen derivatives is a pathologic or a protective response remains to be elucidated.[28]

Clinical Signs of Neonatal Encephalopathy

The clinical manifestations of NE are occasionally apparent immediately or shortly after birth; however, many affected foals are clinically normal at birth and develop clinical signs between 12 and 72 hours of life. Clinical signs range from a mild loss of affinity for the mare and a poorly coordinated suck reflex through to severe CNS dysfunction. Changes in mentation are common and affected foals might alternate between depression or stupor and hyperresponsiveness. Clinical signs are mostly referable to the cerebrum, although some foals also show signs of brain stem or spinal cord dysfunction. Clinical signs commonly include hypotonia, opisthotonus, abnormal respiratory patterns (sometimes leading to hypoxemia and/or hypercapnia), persistent tongue protrusion, and head pressing. Rarely, affected foals vocalize abnormally (hence the colloquial term barker foals). Seizures are common and can range from mild, abnormal movement of the face and jaw to generalized seizures with recumbency and paddling. Interestingly, considering the suggested pathogeneses, the clinical signs of NE can be asymmetric with head tilt, circling behavior, and asymmetric pupillary reflexes commonly described.

Although CNS dysfunction is typically the most obvious clinical sign in foals with NE, other organ systems are often involved and must be considered in the management of these cases. The kidneys and gastrointestinal tract seem to be particularly susceptible but the heart, lungs, liver, adrenal glands, and parathyroid gland can also be affected. In addition to their CNS-related clinical signs, foals with NE often show signs of abnormal gastrointestinal and renal function, including gastric reflux, feeding intolerance, bloat, meconium retention, colic, and persistent increases in creatinine concentration.

Diagnosis

A diagnosis of NE is usually based on the history and presence of appropriate clinical signs in combination with exclusion of other possible differentials. Common differential diagnoses for NE include sepsis, hypoglycemia, and prematurity or dysmaturity. Less common differentials include bacterial meningitis, hydrocephaly, epilepsy, liver disease, viral encephalitis, and toxicosis. Note that foals with NE might also be concurrently septic and/or premature.

Laboratory results might support a diagnosis of NE and can be helpful in detecting comorbidities. Affected foals often have an increased creatinine concentration, perhaps as a consequence of placental insufficiency, but intrinsic renal injury secondary to hypoxia or an inflammatory insult, in addition to altered perfusion or reversion to fetal renal circulation, should also be considered.[47] Low presuckle glucose concentrations have been associated with placental insufficiency, which is recognized as a risk factor for NE.[48,49] Cerebrospinal fluid (CSF) analysis is not commonly performed in foals with NE but can help rule out meningitis. Measurement of the plasma concentrations of neuroactive progestagen derivatives might aid in reaching a diagnosis of NE but these molecules are increased in foals with diseases other than NE. These tests are, therefore, nonspecific but they are also currently not readily available.[39] Although not readily available to most practitioners, measurement of other biomarkers more specifically indicating neurologic injury provides insight into the disorder of NE and might also aid in making a definitive diagnosis.[50] Concentrations of phosphorylated axonal forms of neurofilament H and ubiquitin C-terminal hydrolase 1 are increased in foals with NE compared with normal healthy foals.[50] However, there was some overlap in concentrations between affected foals and healthy foals and this study did not include foals with diseases other than NE.[50]

Electroencephalography (EEG) is used in the management of human neonates with NE or HIE and has the advantage that it can be performed continuously to detect seizure activity.[51,52] EEG background changes are correlated with abnormal findings on MRI of the brain, although the prognostic utility of EEG alone is uncertain. EEG has been described in normal adult horses and foals and a group of adult horses with intracranial disease.[53,54] Changes in the EEG of foals with NE might provide insight into the pathophysiology of the condition and the nature or severity of changes might provide valuable prognostic information, but this has not yet been determined. Performance of EEG in nonsedated or unrestrained foals can be difficult and both sedation and restraint affect recordings.[55] Advanced imaging modalities such as computed tomography (CT) and, particularly, MRI might also provide insight into the pathogenesis of NE but have not been widely used in the management of equine cases. In human infants with HIE, MRI is used to predict long-term neurodevelopmental outcome. At present it is difficult to recommend the routine use of advanced imaging modalities in equine NE cases because the prognosis is typically very good; however, MRI (or CT) might be useful in select cases to rule out other neurologic conditions.[56,57]

Treatment and Management

The treatment of NE in foals is largely supportive and, because the cause of the condition is not completely understood, it is difficult to make definitive treatment recommendations. Treatments for NE have recently been reviewed extensively.[42] What cannot be overemphasized in the care of foals with NE is that excellent nursing care and careful monitoring are essential to ensure optimal outcomes. Clinical experience suggests that foals with NE might be predisposed to sepsis, and many are concurrently septic. Whether this reflects an undiagnosed underlying infectious process, impaired immune function, or increased exposure to pathogens (ie, indiscriminant nursing behavior) is unclear. However, prompt and aggressive broad-spectrum antimicrobial therapy is indicated. Renal function should be carefully monitored, particularly if nephrotoxic antimicrobials are to be administered. Seizure activity increases cerebral oxygen requirements and must be controlled to prevent permanent neurologic injury. Diazepam (0.1–0.4 mg/kg intravenously [IV]) can be used to control occasional or infrequent seizure activity but persistent or frequent seizure activity should be treated with phenobarbital given to effect (begin at 2 mg/kg IV given slowly over

20 minutes; peak effect seen at about 40 minutes after administration; repeat if necessary until control of seizure activity is achieved)[58] or a midazolam constant rate infusion (CRI; 0.02–0.06 mg/kg/h).[59] The advantage of the midazolam CRI is that it allows frequent assessment of neurologic function because midazolam has a very short half-life and can be reversed if necessary.

Tissue perfusion, particularly perfusion of the brain, and arterial oxygenation should be optimized in foals with NE. In many cases this can be achieved with judicious fluid therapy but foals must be carefully monitored to avoid excessive fluid administration. In addition to the risk of tissue edema, many affected foals are unable to excrete the high sodium and chloride load that accompanies (replacement) isotonic, polyionic fluid administration; these foals might require maintenance-type fluids with lower sodium and chloride concentrations and higher potassium concentrations. Foals that are unable to maintain tissue perfusion with fluid administration alone require combinations of inotropes and vasopressors. Arterial oxygenation can be improved in many foals with intranasal oxygen insufflation alone. Foals with respiratory center depression and inadequate respiratory drive can be treated with doxapram (0.02–0.05 mg/kg/h as a CRI), which seems to be more effective than caffeine administration.[60] Foals with persistent or severe hypoxemia and hypercapnia may require short-term mechanical ventilation.

Many foals with NE can tolerate enteral feeding, although it is critical to carefully evaluate their ability to nurse without aspirating. If there is a concern that aspiration might occur, foals can be managed with an indwelling feeding tube. It is important to recognize that sick foals do not need to be fed at the same rate as healthy (growing) foals. The initial aim should be to meet resting energy requirements of sick foals (approximately 50 kcal/kg/d)[61]; increases above this rate should be based on careful monitoring but hyperalimentation can be as deleterious as providing inadequate nutrition. Enteral nutrition is preferred to maintain gastrointestinal function and integrity but some foals are intolerant of enteral nutrition and require some form of parenteral nutrition.

The role of antiinflammatory drugs in the management of NE is unclear, nonsteroidal antiinflammatory drugs are not widely used in human medicine to treat NE and, in the authors' opinion, corticosteroids are not indicated. Pentoxifylline (10 mg/kg by mouth every 12 hours[62]) might suppress tumor necrosis factor alpha expression in adult horses and has been extensively investigated as an antiinflammatory in other species.[63] Studies in rats and other species suggest that pentoxifylline attenuates hypoxic-ischemic injury, although not necessarily of the brain.[64] It should be noted that the bioavailability, appropriate dosage, and efficacy of pentoxifylline have not been examined in the foal. Pharmacologic treatment to stimulate CNS activity and/or reduce neurosteroid concentrations has also been suggested. However, if high neurosteroid concentrations in the neonate are a protective response rather than part of the disorder, attempts to manipulate the concentrations of those molecules are unlikely to improve outcome. A vast array of other treatments have been suggested for the management of NE or HIE, including agents to reduce CNS edema (mannitol, hypertonic saline, dimethyl sulfoxide [DMSO]), free radical scavengers and antioxidants (vitamin E, vitamin C, thiamine [vitamin B_1], DMSO, allopurinol), and NMDA antagonists (magnesium sulfate infusions). Although many of these treatments have a sound theoretic basis, there is limited evidence supporting the efficacy of most.

In contrast, there is considerable evidence supporting the use of hypothermia in the treatment of human brain injury.[65] A recent systematic review that included 11 randomized controlled trials and 1505 infants concluded that therapeutic hypothermia is beneficial in term and late preterm newborns with HIE.[66] Although cooling is associated with some short-term adverse effects, these are thought to be outweighed in human infants by improvements in survival and neurodevelopment. The recommendation of that review was that hypothermia should be instituted in term and late preterm infants with moderate to severe HIE if identified before 6 hours of age.[66] However, it also noted that further trials were required to determine appropriate techniques for cooling neonates and duration of cooling. Because the prognosis for a good outcome in equine neonates with NI is much better than for human infants, advantages of cooling techniques might not be obvious when applied to foals.

Prognosis

Clinical experience and the literature suggest that at least 80% of foals with NE survive and detectable, long-term neurologic deficits seem to be rare. Athletic performance is not expected to be affected in most cases. The presence of sepsis or prematurity likely has a strong influence on outcome in foals concurrently affected by those conditions. It has been proposed that intrauterine growth retardation and NE have implications for many aspects of the long-term health of horses; there is little evidence currently to support this suggestion.[67]

OTHER DISEASES AFFECTING THE NEONATAL EQUINE BRAIN

Conditions that occasionally affect the neonatal equine brain include trauma, bacterial meningitis or meningoencephalitis, cerebellar abiotrophy, and hydrocephalus.

Bacterial infections of the CNS are uncommon in horses but bacterial meningitis and meningoencephalitis are occasionally diagnosed in foals with sepsis.[68–70] The prevalence of bacterial meningitis in septic foals was 5.2% In one recent study but, because the clinical signs are often vague and nonspecific, It is possible that the true prevalence is higher in this population.[69] Organisms isolated from the CSF or CNS tissues include Escherichia coli and Actinobacillus equuli but a wide range of bacteria can be involved. Meningitis has been observed secondary to strangles (Streptococcus equi equi) infection, salmonella diarrhea, vertebral osteomyelitis caused by Rhodococcus equi, and penetrating wounds to the head or neck.[71,72] Clinical signs of bacterial meningitis or meningoencephalitis are variable but include lethargy, weakness, fever, apparent cervical pain, blindness, and seizures. Changes in mentation are invariably described but these can range from mild obtundation to coma. Antemortem confirmation of diagnosis is based on the presence of marked CSF pleocytosis and increased total protein concentration, but these too can be inconsistent. Culture of CSF should be pursued but is often negative. Additional laboratory changes include leukocytosis and an increase in acute phase protein concentrations.[69]

Prognosis for bacterial CNS infection is difficult to predict but is probably poor, with some studies reporting 100% mortality[70]; additionally, residual neurologic deficits have been described in some surviving foals. Achieving effective concentrations of appropriate antimicrobial agents is difficult; some investigators have suggested using third-generation or fourth-generation cephalosporins based on anticipated tissue penetration and sensitivity of bacterial isolates.[69] In human medicine, dexamethasone reportedly improves neurologic outcomes in infants with bacterial meningitis but does not reduce mortality.[73,74]

Cerebellar abiotrophy is familiar to practitioners working with Arabian and Oldenburg horses or Gotland ponies, in which the condition is inherited in certain family lines. Clinical signs might be present at birth but more often develop in the first months of life as a result of cerebellar degeneration. Clinical signs include a wide-based stance; coarse intention tremors of the head; exaggerated responsiveness to stimuli; and a stiff, hypermetric gait affecting all 4 limbs. Although able to see, affected foals never develop a normal menace response.[75] Diagnosis is usually based on clinical signs and signalment; histopathology of the cerebellum reveals degeneration of Purkinje cells and thinning of the molecular and granular layers of the cerebellar cortex.[75]

Hydrocephalus in foals is usually caused by a genetic defect but can also arise secondary to the severe inflammatory response that accompanies meningitis. In either case, there is dilatation of the cerebral ventricles with attenuation of the surrounding tissues. A wide range of nonspecific neurologic signs are described, including altered mentation, poor bonding with the dam, head pressing, compulsive walking, seizures, and the variable development of menace responses. The brain stem is involved in some foals and can result in strabismus or limb ataxia and weakness. Most affected foals are normal in appearance but some have an overly domed appearance to their skulls. The diagnosis of hydrocephalus is usually presumptive but can be confirmed with advanced imaging techniques.

SUMMARY

NE is the most common neurologic condition affecting newborn foals and has often been likened to PAS of human infants. However, in many cases of equine NE there is not an obvious episode of acute hypoxia and most affected foals make a complete recovery, in stark contrast to human infants affected by PAS. In these cases it is possible that foals have experienced chronic hypoxia, perhaps as a result of a placentitis. In addition, clinical experience suggests that in utero infection or inflammation with subsequent exposure to proinflammatory cytokines might be responsible for CNS dysfunction, as has been suggested for some human infants with NE. Increased concentrations of neuroactive progestagens have been found in foals with a clinical diagnosis of NE. Although these molecules might contribute to the clinical signs of neurologic dysfunction, evidence from experimental studies suggests that these neurosteroids may have a protective role.

REFERENCES

1. MacKay RJ. Neurologic disorders of neonatal foals. Vet Clin North Am Equine Pract 2005;21:387–406.
2. Fowden AL, Forhead AJ, Ousey JC. Endocrine adaptations in the foal over the perinatal period. Equine Vet J Suppl 2012;(41):130–9.
3. Fowden AL, Forhead AJ, Ousey JC. The Endocrinology of equine parturition. Exp Clin Endocrinol Diabetes 2008;116:393–403.
4. Chavatte P, Holtan D, Ousey JC, et al. Biosynthesis and possible biological roles of progestagens during equine pregnancy and in the newborn foal. Equine Vet J Suppl 1997;(24):89–95.
5. Silver M. Placental progestagens in the sheep and horse and the changes leading to parturition. Exp Clin Endocrinol 1994;102:203–11.
6. Ousey JC. Peripartal endocrinology in the mare and foetus. Reprod Domest Anim 2004;39:222–31.
7. Silver M. Prenatal maturation, the timing of birth and how it may be regulated in domestic animals. Exp Physiol 1990;75:285–307.
8. Sangild PT, Fowden AL, Trahair JF. How does the foetal gastrointestinal tract develop in preparation for enteral nutrition after birth? Livest Prod Sci 2000;66: 141–50.

9. Gold JR, Cohen ND, Welsh TH Jr. Association of adrenocorticotrophin and cortisol concentrations with peripheral blood leukocyte cytokine gene expression in septic and nonseptic neonatal foals. J Vet Intern Med 2012;26:654–61.

10. Gold JR, Divers TJ, Barton MH, et al. Plasma adrenocorticotropin, cortisol, and adrenocorticotropin/cortisol ratios in septic and normal-term foals. J Vet Intern Med 2007;21:791–6.

11. Hart KA, Slovis NM, Barton MH. Hypothalamic-pituitary-adrenal axis dysfunction in hospitalized neonatal foals. J Vet Intern Med 2009;23:901–12.

12. Hurcombe SDA, Toribio RE, Slovis N, et al. Blood arginine vasopressin, adrenocorticotropin hormone, and cortisol concentrations at admission in septic and critically ill foals and their association with survival. J Vet Intern Med 2008;22:639–47.

13. Mellon SH, Griffin LD. Neurosteroids: biochemistry and clinical significance. Trends Endocrinol Metab 2002;13:35–43.

14. Crossley KJ, Nicol MB, Hirst JJ, et al. Suppression of arousal by progesterone in fetal sheep. Reprod Fertil Dev 1997;9:767–73.

15. Crossley KJ, Nitsos I, Walker DW, et al. Steroid-sensitive GABA(A) receptors in the fetal sheep brain. Neuropharmacology 2003;45:461–72.

16. Belelli D, Herd MB, Mitchell EA, et al. Neuroactive steroids and inhibitory neurotransmission: mechanisms of action and physiological relevance. Neuroscience 2006;138:821–9.

17. Lambert JJ, Belelli D, Peden DR, et al. Neurosteroid modulation of GABAA receptors. Prog Neurobiol 2003;71:67–80.

18. Diesch TJ, Mellor DJ. Birth transitions: pathophysiology, the onset of consciousness and possible implications for neonatal maladjustment syndrome in the foal. Equine Vet J 2013;45:656–60.

19. Holtan DW, Houghton E, Silver M, et al. Plasma progestagens in the mare, fetus and newborn foal. J Reprod Fertil Suppl 1991;44:517–28.

20. Hirst JJ, Kelleher MA, Walker DW, et al. Neuroactive steroids in pregnancy: key regulatory and protective roles in the foetal brain. J Steroid Biochem Mol Biol 2014;139:144–53.

21. Nicol MB, Hirst JJ, Walker D, et al. Effect of alteration of maternal plasma progesterone concentrations on fetal behavioural state during late gestation. J Endocrinol 1997;152:379–86.

22. Nicol MB, Hirst JJ, Walker DW. Effect of pregnane steroids on electrocortical activity and somatosensory evoked potentials in fetal sheep. Neurosci Lett 1998; 253:111–4.

23. Nicol MB, Hirst JJ, Walker DW. Effect of finasteride on behavioural arousal and somatosensory evoked potentials in fetal sheep. Neurosci Lett 2001;306:13–6.

24. Yawno T, Hirst JJ, Castillo-Melendez M, et al. Role of neurosteroids in regulating cell death and proliferation in the late gestation fetal brain. Neuroscience 2009; 163:838–47.

25. Schumacher M, Guennoun R, Robert F, et al. Local synthesis and dual actions of progesterone in the nervous system: neuroprotection and myelination. Growth Hormone & IGF Research 2004;(14 Suppl A):S18–33.

26. Hirst JJ, Yawno T, Nguyen P, et al. Stress in pregnancy activates neurosteroid production in the fetal brain. Neuroendocrinology 2006;84:264–74.

27. Nguyen PN, Yan EB, Castillo-Melendez M, et al. Increased allopregnanolone levels in the fetal sheep brain following umbilical cord occlusion. J Physiol 2004;560:593–602.

28. Hirst JJ, Palliser HK, Yates DM, et al. Neurosteroids in the fetus and neonate: potential protective role in compromised pregnancies. Neurochem Int 2008;52:602–10.

29. Billiards SS, Nguyen PN, Scheerlinck JP, et al. Hypoxia potentiates endotoxin-induced allopregnanolone concentrations in the newborn brain. Biol Neonate 2006;90:258–67.
30. Billiards SS, Walker DW, Canny BJ, et al. Endotoxin increases sleep and brain allopregnanolone concentrations in newborn lambs. Pediatr Res 2002;52:892–9.
31. Bucolo C, Drago F. Effects of neurosteroids on ischemia-reperfusion injury in the rat retina: role of sigma (1) recognition sites. Eur J Pharmacol 2004;498:111–4.
32. Djebaili M, Guo QM, Pettus EH, et al. The neurosteroids progesterone and allopregnanolone reduce cell death, gliosis, and functional deficits after traumatic brain injury in rats. J Neurotrauma 2005;22:106–18.
33. Frank C, Sagratella S. Neuroprotective effects of allopregnenolone on hippocampal irreversible neurotoxicity in vitro. Prog Neuropsychopharmacol Biol Psychiatry 2000;24:1117–26.
34. Nicol MB, Hirst JJ, Walker D. Effects of pregnanolone on behavioural parameters and the responses to GABA(A) receptor antagonists in the late gestation fetal sheep. Neuropharmacology 1999;38:49–63.
35. Yawno T, Yan EB, Walker DW, et al. Inhibition of neurosteroid synthesis increases asphyxia-induced brain injury in the late gestation fetal sheep. J Soc Gynecol Investig 2006;13:73a–4a.
36. Nguyen PN, Billiards SS, Walker DW, et al. Changes in 5 alpha-pregnane steroids and neurosteroidogenic enzyme expression in fetal sheep with umbilicoplacental embolization. Pediatr Res 2003;54:840–7.
37. Houghton E, Holtan D, Grainger L, et al. Plasma progestagen concentrations in the normal and dysmature newborn foal. J Reprod Fertil 1991;44:609–17.
38. Rossdale PD, Ousey JC, Mcgladdery AJ, et al. A retrospective study of increased plasma progestagen concentrations in compromised neonatal foals. Reprod Fertil Dev 1995;7:567–75.
39. Aleman M, Pickles KJ, Conley AJ, et al. Abnormal plasma neuroactive progestagen derivatives in ill, neonatal foals presented to the neonatal intensive care unit. Equine Vet J 2013;45:661–5.
40. Madigan JE, Haggett EF, Pickles KJ, et al. Allopregnanolone infusion induced neurobehavioural alterations in a neonatal foal: is this a clue to the pathogenesis of neonatal maladjustment syndrome? Equine Vet J 2012;44:109–12.
41. Palmer AC, Rossdale PD. Neuropathological changes associated with neonatal maladjustment syndrome in thoroughbred foal. Res Vet Sci 1976;20:267–75.
42. Wong D, Wilkins PA, Bain FT, et al. Neonatal encephalopathy in foals. Compend Contin Educ Vet 2011;33:E5.
43. McAuliffe JJ, Miles L, Vorhees CV. Adult neurological function following neonatal hypoxia-ischemia in a mouse model of the term neonate: water maze performance is dependent on separable cognitive and motor components. Brain Res 2006;1118:208–21.
44. van Handel M, Swaab H, de Vries LS, et al. Long-term cognitive and behavioral consequences of neonatal encephalopathy following perinatal asphyxia: a review. Eur J Pediatr 2007;166:645–54.
45. Viscardi RM, Muhumuza CK, Rodriguez A, et al. Inflammatory markers in intrauterine and fetal blood and cerebrospinal fluid compartments are associated with adverse pulmonary and neurologic outcomes in preterm infants. Pediatr Res 2004;55:1009–17.
46. Shalak LF, Laptook AR, Jafri HS, et al. Clinical chorioamnionitis, elevated cytokines, and brain injury in term infants. Pediatrics 2002;110:673–80.

47. Chaney KP, Holcombe SJ, Schott HC 2nd, et al. Spurious hypercreatininemia: 28 neonatal foals (2000-2008). J Vet Emerg Crit Care (San Antonio) 2010;20:244–9.
48. Vaala WE. Peripartum asphyxia. Vet Clin North Am Equine Pract 1994;10: 187–218.
49. Furr M. Perinatal asphyxia in foals. Compend Contin Educ Vet 1996;18:1342–51.
50. Ringger NC, Giguere S, Morresey PR, et al. Biomarkers of brain injury in foals with hypoxic-ischemic encephalopathy. J Vet Intern Med 2011;25:132–7.
51. El-Ayouty M, Abdel-Hady H, El-Mogy S, et al. Relationship between electroencephalography and magnetic resonance imaging findings after hypoxic-ischemic encephalopathy at term. Am J Perinatol 2007;24:467–73.
52. Nanavati T, Seemaladinne N, Regier M, et al. Can we predict functional outcome in neonates with hypoxic ischemic encephalopathy by the combination of neuroimaging and electroencephalography? Pediatr Neonatol 2015. http://dx.doi.org/10.1016/j.pedneo.2014.12.005.
53. Lacombe VA, Podell M, Furr M, et al. Diagnostic validity of electroencephalography in equine intracranial disorders. J Vet Intern Med 2001;15:385–93.
54. Mysinger PW, Redding RW, Vaughan JT, et al. Electroencephalographic patterns of clinically normal, sedated, and tranquilized newborn foals and adult horses. Am J Vet Res 1985;46:36–41.
55. Toth B, Aleman M, Brosnan RJ, et al. Evaluation of squeeze-induced somnolence in neonatal foals. Am J Vet Res 2012;73:1881–9.
56. Chaffin MK, Walker MA, McArthur NH, et al. Magnetic resonance imaging of the brain of normal neonatal foals. Vet Radiol Ultrasound 1997;38:102–11.
57. Ferrell EA, Gavin PR, Tucker RL, et al. Magnetic resonance for evaluation of neurologic disease in 12 horses. Vet Radiol Ultrasound 2002;43:510–6.
58. Wilkins P. Disorders of foals. In: Reed S, Bayly W, Sellon D, editors. Equine internal medicine. 2nd edition. St Louis (MO): Saunders; 2004. p. 1381–430.
59. Wilkins P. How to use midazolam to control equine neonatal seizures. AAEP Annual Convention; 2005. p. 279–80.
60. Giguere S, Slade JK, Sanchez LC. Retrospective comparison of caffeine and doxapram for the treatment of hypercapnia in foals with hypoxic-ischemic encephalopathy. J Vet Intern Med 2008;22:401–5.
61. Jose-Cunilleras E, Viu J, Corradini I, et al. Energy expenditure of critically ill neonatal foals. Equine Vet J Suppl 2012;(41):48–51.
62. Liska DA, Akucewich LH, Marsella R, et al. Pharmacokinetics of pentoxifylline and its 5-hydroxyhexyl metabolite after oral and intravenous administration of pentoxifylline to healthy adult horses. Am J Vet Res 2006;67:1621–7.
63. Barton MH, Ferguson D, Davis PJ, et al. The effects of pentoxifylline infusion on plasma 6-keto-prostaglandin F1 alpha and ex vivo endotoxin-induced tumour necrosis factor activity in horses. J Vet Pharmacol Ther 1997;20:487–92.
64. Kalay S, Islek A, Ozturk A, et al. Pentoxifylline therapy attenuates intestinal injury in rat pups with hypoxic ischemic encephalopathy. J Matern Fetal Neonatal Med 2014;27:1476–80.
65. Srinivasakumar P, Zempel J, Wallendorf M, et al. Therapeutic hypothermia in neonatal hypoxic ischemic encephalopathy: electrographic seizures and magnetic resonance imaging evidence of injury. J Pediatr 2013;163:465–70.
66. Jacobs SE, Berg M, Hunt R, et al. Cooling for newborns with hypoxic ischaemic encephalopathy. Cochrane Database Syst Rev 2013;(1):CD003311.
67. Ousey JC, Rossdale PD, Fowden AL, et al. Effects of manipulating intrauterine growth on post natal adrenocortical development and other parameters of maturity in neonatal foals. Equine Vet J 2004;36:616–21.

68. Toth B, Aleman M, Nogradi N, et al. Meningitis and meningoencephalomyelitis in horses: 28 cases (1985-2010). J Am Vet Med Assoc 2012;240:580–7.
69. Viu J, Monreal L, Jose-Cunilleras E, et al. Clinical findings in 10 foals with bacterial meningoencephalitis. Equine Vet J Suppl 2012;(41):100–4.
70. Sanchez LC, Giguere S, Lester GD. Factors associated with survival of neonatal foals with bacteremia and racing performance of surviving thoroughbreds: 423 cases (1982-2007). J Am Vet Med Assoc 2008;233:1446–52.
71. Finno C, Pusterla N, Aleman M, et al. *Streptococcus equi* meningoencephalomyelitis in a foal. J Am Vet Med Assoc 2006;229:721–4.
72. Smith JJ, Provost PJ, Paradis MR. Bacterial meningitis and brain abscesses secondary to infectious disease processes involving the head in horses: seven cases (1980-2001). J Am Vet Med Assoc 2004;224:739–42.
73. Mongelluzzo J, Mohamad Z, Ten Have TR, et al. Corticosteroids and mortality in children with bacterial meningitis. JAMA 2008;299:2048–55.
74. Brouwer MC, McIntyre P, Prasad K, et al. Corticosteroids for acute bacterial meningitis. Cochrane Database Syst Rev 2013;(6):CD004405.
75. Palmer AC, Blakemore WF, Cook WR, et al. Cerebellar hypoplasia and degeneration in the young Arab horse: clinical and neuropathological features. Vet Rec 1973;93:62–6.

The Normal and Abnormal Equine Neonatal Musculoskeletal System

David G. Levine, DVM

KEYWORDS

- Musculoskeletal • Ossification • Synovial infection • Osteomyelitis • Flexural limb
- Angular limb

KEY POINTS

- The first few weeks of life are critical in horses.
- Cuboidal bone ossification at birth can vary and should be assessed in premature and dysmature foals.
- Flexural limb deformities, angular limb deformity, and laxity are common in neonatal foals and should be assessed and treated early.
- Neonatal foals are susceptible to septic orthopedic conditions owing to immature immune system and physeal blood flow. Early recognition and treatment is key to success.

NORMAL OSSIFICATION

In the typical foal, the tarsal and carpal bones ossify in the last 2 to 3 months of gestation.[1] The normal process of endochondrial ossification starts centrally within the bone and the process continues until the periphery of the bone is mature with the normal surrounding cartilage. Ossification of the cuboidal bones plays an important role in the foal, but should not be confused with total skeletal maturity.[2] In the human, skeletal maturity is determined by radiographs of the axial skeleton because cuboidal bones are not a reliable index for total skeletal maturity.[3,4]

A skeletal ossification index has been used to standardize the evaluation of newborn foals.[2] The index is based on 2 radiographic views of the carpus and tarsus, and 4 grades have been developed.

- Grade 1: Some of the cuboidal bones of the carpus and tarsus have no radiographic evidence of ossification (**Fig. 1**).
- Grade 2: Some radiographic evidence of ossification of all of the cuboidal bones of the carpus and tarsus (excluding the first carpal bone). The proximal physes of the third metacarpus/metatarsus were open (**Fig. 2**).

University of Pennsylvania, New Bolton Center, 382 W. Street Road, Kennett Square, PA 19348, USA
E-mail address: dglevine@vet.upenn.edu

Vet Clin Equine 31 (2015) 601–613
http://dx.doi.org/10.1016/j.cveq.2015.09.003
0749-0739/15/$ – see front matter © 2015 Elsevier Inc. All rights reserved.
vetequine.theclinics.com

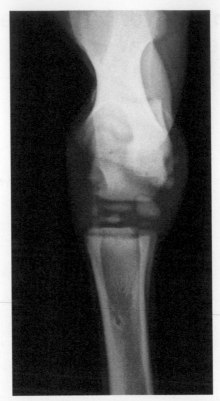

Fig. 1. Grade 1 ossification. Some of the cuboidal bones show no evidence of ossification.

- Grade 3: All of the cuboidal bones were ossified, but they were small with rounded edges. The joint spaces thus seemed to be wide in these individuals. The lateral styloid process and the malleoli were distinct. The proximal physes of the third metacarpus and metatarsus were closed (**Fig. 3**).

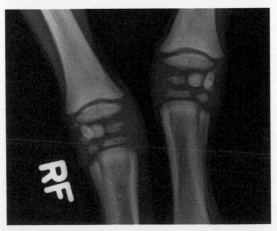

Fig. 2. Grade 2 ossification. All cuboidal bones have some evidence of ossification. There is a faint line representing the open proximal metacarpal physes.

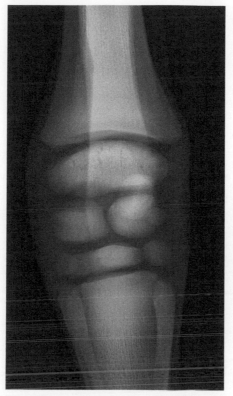

Fig. 3. Grade 3 ossification. All cuboidal bones are present but have rounded edges with increased joint space and the proximal metacarpal physis is closed.

- Grade 4: All of the criteria of grade 3 were met, and the cuboidal bones were shaped like the corresponding bones in the adult and the joint spaces were of expected width (**Fig. 4**).

A common condition in immature foals is incomplete ossification of the cuboidal bones. This condition is not limited to the immature foal; dysmature foals may also display this condition. There are many reported causes for incomplete ossification of the cuboidal bones. These can include[1,5,6]:

- Prematurity related to short gestational age (<320 days);
- Dysmaturity secondary to placentitis;
- Placental insufficiency;
- Fetal infection;
- Severe, prolonged metabolic disturbances (maternal malnutrition);
- Twin foals;
- Heavy parasitism that may decrease blood supply to the uterus;
- Colic or shock in the mare, which may alter the blood supply to the fetus and retard its growth;
- Vaccinations and anthelmintics administered during pregnancy that could influence development; and
- Thyroid abnormalities that could retard ossification.[5]

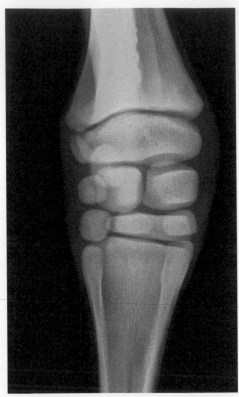

Fig. 4. Grade 4 ossification. All cuboidal bones are normally shaped and the joint spaces are normal.

Although more severe cases may show signs of angular deformity or a broken tarsal axis, many can go unnoticed. Because foals have some natural angular deformity of the carpus (carpal valgus) at birth, weight is not evenly distributed across the carpus. This uneven stress along with the softer cartilaginous precursor of normal bone can lead to deformity of the lateral bones in the carpus (ulnar, intermediate, and third and fourth carpal bones). In the tarsus, the stresses are in a sagittal plane and deformity of the cranial aspect of the cuboidal bones (central and third tarsal bones). For this reason, it is important to diagnose the condition early.

Treatment for incomplete ossification depends on the severity of the condition. Stall rest and exercise restriction can be used for foals with incomplete ossification of the carpi and straight limbs. No turnout or exercise should be permitted until complete ossification has occurred, because this can lead to permanent damage of the ossifying cartilage and the development of osteoarthritis. Depending on the level of immaturity or dysmaturity, complete ossification should occur within 4 weeks. Radiographs should be taken every other week during this time.

For foals with incomplete ossification with limbs that are not straight, or for incomplete ossification of the tarsus, treatment should include external splints or casts. The goal of external coaptation is to maintain the limb in proper alignment and prevent damage to the developing bone. The splints or casts should not include the foot and should stop above the fetlock joint. If the foot is incorporated in the splint, the musculotendinous flexor and extensor units weaken, resulting in a dropped fetlock and osteopenia. Splints should be changed every 3 to 4 days, and dry padding is placed next to the limb. Casts should be changed between 10 and 14 days. Care should be taken to prevent pressure sores over the point of the hock as well as the accessory carpal bone. A downside of external coaptation is the resulting laxity from immobilization of the flexor and extensor tendons. This condition is temporary and controlled exercise after removal improves strength. To avoid this complication, many custom braces are now available that allow movement of the limb while maintaining alignment. These custom braces can be expensive, but can decrease laxity thus allowing a more rapid return to function after ossification.[7]

FLEXURAL LIMB DEFORMITIES

Flexural limb deformities can be defined as a deviation from the normal sagittal plane when viewed from the side. It manifests clinically as an inability to extend the limb fully. Although classically called "contracted tendons," this is a misnomer. More accurately, it is a difference in the length of the bone versus the soft tissue structures. This can include the digital flexor tendons, the suspensory apparatus (including suspensory ligament and distal sesamoidean ligaments), as well as the joint capsule and surrounding fascia. In some cases, bony deformation of the bones and joints also occurs. Severe flexural limb deformities can be a cause of dystocia in the mare, which can lead to loss of both mare and foal. We limit our discussion to the congenital flexural deformities that occur at birth.

There are many suspected causes of congenital flexural deformities. Although there is limited proof of these causes, they include[8–10]:

- In utero malposition;
- Genetic predisposition;
- Poor nutrition; and
- Exposure to teratogens.

Congenital flexural limb deformities most commonly affect the carpus, tarsus, metacarpophalangeal, metatarsophalangeal, and distal interphalangeal joints.[8–10] Severity can range from mild contracture to an inability of the foal to stand and nurse. Diagnosis can be made after parturition with visual and physical examination of the foal both recumbent and standing. If severe deformities are noted, radiographic examination is warranted to determine whether congenital bone deformation has occurred.

Treatment depends on the severity of the condition as well as the structures involved. Severe cases with a palmar angle of less than 90°, associated bone deformation, or other congenital abnormalities (wry nose, spinal deformation) should in most cases be humanely euthanized. There are, however, some case reports where these foals have survived with surgical intervention with limited to no athletic potential.[8,11,12] Options for treatment can include 1 or more of the following.

- Physiotherapy: This can be performed by manually extending the limb in 10 to 15 minute therapy sessions 4 to 6 times daily. This therapy works best for mild flexural deformities and can be done with the foal recumbent (often while resting after nursing) or while standing and forced to ambulate on the limb.
- Bandaging: Bandages can be applied to the limb to create laxity of the joints. This works well for mild to moderate cases. For carpal and tarsal contracture where the distal limb is normal, the bandages can end above the metacarpophalangeal/metatarsophalangeal joint to avoid laxity of the distal limb. Care must be taken to change bandages often (every other day or more) to look for pressure

sores that can develop quickly in areas of high pressure (usually along dorsal aspect of contracted area).

- Rubber bands: Using rubber bands (IV simplex tubing) over bandages on the dorsal aspect of the limb can aid in physical therapy without the complications seen with splinting. This is done by lightly bandaging the limb followed by attaching a stretched out rubber band over the dorsal aspect of the limb to apply constant extension pressure on the limb (**Fig. 5**).
- Splinting: Splints are commonly used in more moderate cases to hasten straightening of the limb. Splints can be made of many types of materials (PVC, cast tape, commercial splints custom made for foals). Splints should be applied over light bandages and changed often to avoid pressure sores, which are more common when splinting compared with bandaging. Splints can be used intermittently during the day with 6 hours on and 6 hours off to avoid pressure sores. It may also be beneficial to sedate the foal while applying the splints to aid in straightening the limb. The splints should be bent for use over the metacarpophalangeal/metatarsophalangeal joint to achieve dorsiflexion of the joints.
- Casting: Casting can be used in moderate cases of flexural limb deformities. Casts are applied soon after parturition and changed in 24 to 48 hours. Substantial improvement should be seen after 1 to 2 cast applications. Casts decrease the labor needed to change splints every 4 to 6 hours and decrease pressure

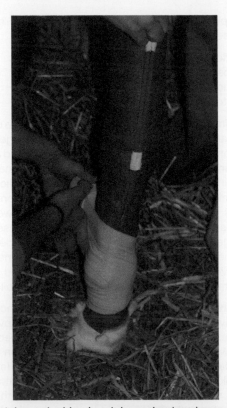

Fig. 5. Placement of a tightened rubber band down the dorsal aspect of the limb. The band is attached to the toe and then stretched and wrapped with an adhesive elastic bandage.

sores. Foals that are in bilateral splints or casts often need assistance standing and nursing, and should be housed in a facility that has 24-hour intensive care.

- Oxytetracycline: Intravenous oxytetracycline has been used to induce laxity in foals affected with flexural limb deformities.[13] The mechanism is not understood clearly, but it seems to be more beneficial in younger foals (first 2 weeks of life). The dose commonly used is 44 mg/kg (2–4 g) given slowly intravenously. This is a larger dose than commonly used in adults. Some foals can develop renal failure from oxytetracycline administration and an evaluation of serum creatinine is recommended before administration. This dose can be repeated once daily for 2 to 3 days and used in combination with splinting and bandaging. Besides renal toxicity, some foals can develop diarrhea as well as laxity of other joints after administration.[9,10]

- Surgery: Surgery is not recommended commonly for congenital flexural deformities and is more common for acquired deformities. Surgical intervention including superior and inferior check desmotomy can be used to aid in laxity **(Fig. 6)**. In more severe cases of flexural deformity, cutting of the flexor tendons and palmar carpal ligaments, as well as the joint capsule and soft tissues, has been used to save foals. Other cases of bone deformation and arthrogryposis have been saved with invasive surgical techniques, including arthrodesis and plating techniques.[11,12]

Prognosis depends on the severity of the flexural deformity. If the foal is able to stand, nurse, and ambulate, the prognosis is favorable with treatment. Foals that respond in the first 2 weeks have the best prognosis for athletic performance, although some cases of carpal contracture can take longer to respond. Severe deformities where the foal is unable to stand and where bone deformation has occurred have a poor prognosis. Early recognition is critical because foals that are sore owing to

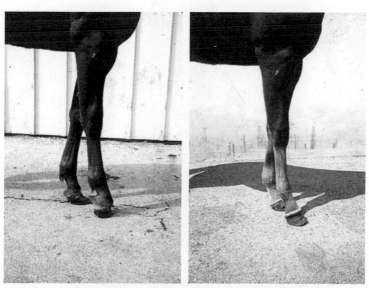

Fig. 6. Right forelimb of a foal before (*left*) and after (*right*) inferior check desmotomy. Note the severity of the flexural deformity that prompted surgical intervention over conservative treatment.

flexural deformities will not use the limb. This disuse will increase the flexural deformity and make treatment more difficult.

Laxity

Neonatal foals are often born with some degree of tendon and ligament laxity. This is more common in the hind limbs than the forelimbs. This laxity of the distal limb causes increased dorsiflexion of the metacarpo/metatarsophalangeal joint and distal interphalangeal joints. In more severe cases, the palmar/plantar aspect of the fetlock or the heel bulbs may touch the ground (**Fig. 7**). Most cases correct within days but some more advanced cases do require treatment.

Treatment

- Controlled exercise: Walking the foal with the mare strengthens the musculotendinous unit and improvement should be noted quickly (within a few days).
- Bandaging: Bandages are often applied by inexperienced owners to protect and "support" the limb. Unfortunately, bandaging causes increased laxity and should be avoided. If some protection is needed to the palmar/plantar aspect of the fetlock, padding with limited bandaging should be used.
- Shoeing/trimming: Application of a heel extension can aid in support of the distal limb and can be used in more severe cases.

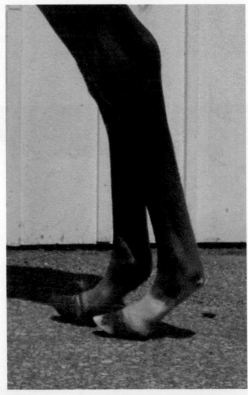

Fig. 7. Moderate tendon laxity in a foal. Note the small abrasion on the plantar aspect of the metatarsophalangeal joint.

ANGULAR LIMB DEFORMITY

Angular limb deformity is defined as deviation from the long axis of the limb in the frontal plane. This can either be a varus deformity (medial deviation of the limb distal to the deformity) or a valgus deformity (lateral deviation of the limb distal to the deformity). Foals are often born with a mild carpal valgus deviation, which is considered normal. Although angular deformities are often lumped together with concurrent rotational deformity (toed-out with valgus, pigeon toed with varus) these are separate rotation defects that should be noted. An external rotation of the front limbs (toed-out) is normal in neonatal foals and will correct as the chest of the foal expands and the limbs naturally rotate inward.

Diagnosis of congenital angular limb deformities should be done with the foal standing and ambulating toward and away from the observer. It is important to look at each limb from the dorsal and palmar/plantar aspect of the limb and not from the front/back of the foal. The external and internal rotation of the limb can make the limb seem angular when it is in fact normal (**Fig. 8**). In more severe cases, radiographs can be used to measure the angle of the deformity and for surgical planning.

Most causes of congenital angular limb deformity are related to periarticular laxity or incomplete ossification (see Laxity). Cases of periarticular laxity are most commonly self-limiting. Foals should be treated conservatively with stall rest and limited exercise and resolution is usually seen in the first 2 to 4 weeks of life. This can be seen commonly in windswept foals, where 1 limb demonstrates a varus deformity and the other limb demonstrates a valgus deformity that corrects itself. Bandaging,

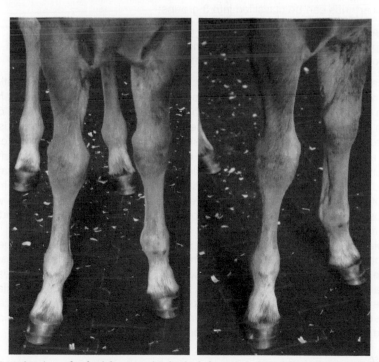

Fig. 8. Examination of a foal for angular limb deformity looking from the front of the foal (*left*) and the frontal plane (front of limb, *right*). This demonstrates the importance of looking at the limb from its frontal plane.

splinting, and casting are not recommended for periarticular laxity because it will increase the laxity of the joint and compound the problem.

More moderate to severe cases of congenital angular deformity are also seen. Surgical intervention is rarely needed in the first 2 weeks of life, although severe deformity of the fetlock region should be evaluated in the first month. Growth plate closure of the radius and tibia afford longer time for conservative management. In severe cases of angular deformity where the foal is unable to bear weight normally, glue-on shoes can be used to aid in ambulation.

ORTHOPEDIC SEPSIS

The neonatal foal's immune system is associated mainly with passively acquired immunity. The rapid decrease in passive antibodies mixed with the slow rise of the foals immune system make foals more susceptible to infections.[14] Failure of passive transfer can occur by inadequate intake of colostrum, poor quality colostrum, or inadequate absorption of antibodies.[15] Septic arthritis is a common consequence of bacteremia and septicemia in foals. It can account for 12% of mortality in the first month of life.[16]

Neonatal foals have unique blood supply that predisposes localization of bacteria to the joints. Transphyseal vessels bring blood across from the metaphysis to the epiphysis, which allows bacteria easier access to the joint. The synovial cavity is a perfect place for bacteria to thrive with limited natural host defense mechanisms and decreased blood flow, limiting the host response to infection. These vessels normally close in the first 2 weeks of life, which can change the location of infection depending on the timing of sepsis.

Septic arthritis can be classified into 3 groups:

- Type S: septic arthritis with no bone involvement;
- Type E: osteomyelitis of the subchondral bone plate and epiphysis; and
- Type P: osteomyelitis of the physis at the metaphyseal junction.

Clinical signs can vary based on the location of the infection. Septic arthritis clinically can start with mild edema over the joint with rapid progression to joint effusion. Effusion can be severe and can be noted before the onset of lameness. Often owners note the swelling and assume the foal suffered external trauma, although this is rarely the case. The pressure caused by the effusion along with inflammatory mediators lead to pain and lameness. Foals with type P osteomyelitis may not have joint effusion, depending on whether the physeal infection enters the joint. These foals may have localized swelling and pain over the physis and can drain locally without joint involvement. Often this occurs in foals over 2 weeks of age after the transphyseal vessels have closed and hematogenous bacteria localize within the rapidly growing and highly vascularized physis.

Inoculation of bone instead of synovial structures is also possible in the neonatal foal. It can often be more difficult to determine the cause of lameness in these foals because the radiographic change can occur days after the onset of lameness with no visual swelling over the bone affected. Cases where inoculation of the axial skeleton are involved can prove to be the most difficult to diagnose. In acute cases of lameness in the neonatal foal, sepsis of synovial structures as well as bone should always be on the differential list and be ruled out.

Diagnosis

The most common clinical sign of orthopedic infection is lameness. This may occur after a systemic septic event, although many times the systemic event is not recognized clinically. Increased rectal temperature is variable. Routine bloodwork may show an increase in peripheral white blood cell counts, although this is not reliable. Serum fibrinogen concentration is often increased in foals with orthopedic sepsis and fibrinogen concentrations of more than 1000 mg/dL are suggestive of bone involvement.[17] Serum amyloid A is also a useful in acute cases of orthopedic sepsis. Unlike fibrinogen, serum amyloid A increases more rapidly in cases of sepsis and can be used serially to determine response to treatment. More data on the use of serum amyloid A are needed, but the fast response time and shorter half-life of this acute phase protein make it more ideal than fibrinogen in looking at acute infections.

Arthrocentesis of effusive joints should be performed. Because many cases of synovial sepsis involve more than 1 joint, it is important to palpate all joints and sample all those that have any clinical suspicion of effusion. High total protein concentrations (>2 g/dL) and high leukocyte counts (>10,000 cells/μL; primarily neutrophils) are typical. Foals with septic synovial structures can often have leukocyte counts of greater than 50,000 cells/μL, although cell count does not seem to correspond with the severity of disease.[18,19] Samples should be submitted for culture and sensitivity, often accompanied with a blood culture, to determine whether systemic sepsis is an ongoing problem. A complete physical examination looking for other sources of sepsis (lungs, gastrointestinal, umbilical) should always be performed.

Radiographs should be obtained of affected joints to determine physeal and metaphyseal involvement. In early cases, these radiographs can serve as a baseline to follow-up examinations. Radiographic change often lags behind the clinical picture and bone that seems to be normal radiographically may still be affected.

Treatment

Treatment should consist of aggressive local and, if indicated, systemic antimicrobial therapy. Broad-spectrum antimicrobials are commonly started until a positive culture or clinical suspicion helps to guide antimicrobial choice. Lavage of the septic structures can be done with through-and-through needle lavage or more aggressively with an arthrotomy or arthroscopy. Several studies have shown the benefit of more aggressive treatment with arthotomy/arthroscopy with improved survival and no increase in morbidity.[19,20] This is owing to the removal of fibrin, inflammatory mediators, and diseased bone and synovial membrane that cannot be removed by simple needle lavage. Local implantation of antibiotic impregnated beads, intraarticular injection of antimicrobials, and regional limb perfusions can be used in addition to lavage and may improve the outcome.[20] Although regional limb perfusion is an appropriate way to deliver high concentrations of antimicrobials to the distal limb, intraarticular injections still achieve higher concentrations within the joint as well as adjacent bone.

Prognosis

Survival in these cases ranges from 45% to 85%.[21] Athletic outcome depends on the number of joints affected, severity of infection, as well as the response to treatment. Thoroughbred foals have been shown to have a decreased likelihood to race compared with controls with only 30% of survivors becoming racehorses.[22,23] Factors that decrease survival include[21–23]:

- Duration of infection before treatment;
- Number of joints affected;
- Bone involvement; and
- Multisystemic disease.

SUMMARY

The first weeks of a foal's life can be challenging. Orthopedic conditions can occur frequently and some do require emergency treatment. The key is early diagnosis and appropriate care. Prognosis for most conditions improves with early recognition and corrective treatments. It is important to know the appropriate treatment for each condition because often the incorrect treatment can lead to further complications.

REFERENCES

1. McIlwraith CW. Incomplete ossification of carpal and tarsal bones in foals. Equine Vet Ed 2003;15(2):79–81.
2. Adams R, Poulos P. A skeletal ossification index for neonatal foals. Vet Radiol 1988;29:217–22.
3. Kuhns LR, Finnstrom O. New standards of ossification of the newborn. Radiology 1976;119:655–60.
4. Kuhns LR, Sherman MP, Poznanski AK. Determination of neonatal maturation on the chest radiograph. Radiology 1972;102:597–603.
5. Auer JA, Martens RJ, Morris EL. Angular limb deformities in foals. Comp Cont Educ Pract Vet 1982;4:330–9.
6. Rossdale PD, Ousey JC. Fetal programming for athletic performance in the horse: potential effects of IUGR. Equine Vet Ed 2002;14:98–112.
7. Auer J. Angular limb deformities. In: Auer JA, editor. Equine surgery. St Louis (MO): Elsevier; 2012. p. 1201–21.
8. Hunt RJ. Flexural limb deformities. In: Ross MW, Dyson SJ, editors. Diagnosis and management of lameness in the horse. St Louis (MO): Elsevier; 2003. p. 562–5.
9. Adams SB, Santschi EM. Management of flexural limb deformities in young horses. Equine Pract 1999;21:9–16.
10. Auer JA. Flexural limb deformities. In: Auer JA, editor. Equine surgery. St Louis (MO): Elsevier; 2012. p. 1150–65.
11. Adams SB, Santschi EM. Management of congenital and acquired flexural limb deformities. Proceedings AAEP 2000;46:117–25.
12. Whitehair KJ, Adams SB, Toombs JP, et al. Arthrodesis for congenital flexural deformity of the metacarpophalangeal and metatarsophalangeal joints. Vet Surg 1992;22:228–33.
13. Madison JB, Garber JL, Rice B, et al. Effect of oxytetracycline on metacarpophalangeal and distal interphalangeal joint angles in new born foals. J Am Vet Med Assoc 1994;204:240–9.
14. Trumble TN. Orthopedic disorders in neonatal foals. Vet Clin Equine 2005;21: 357–85.
15. Stoneham SJ, Digby NJ, Ricketts SW. Failure of passive transfer of colostral immunity in the foal. Vet Rec 1991;22:42–5.
16. Cohen ND. Causes of and farm management factors associated with disease and death in foals. J Am Vet Med Assoc 1994;204:1644–51.
17. Madison JB, Sommer M, Spencer PA. Relations among synovial membrane histopathologic findings, synovial fluid cytologic findings, and bacterial culture results in horses with suspected infectious arthritis. J Am Vet Med Assoc 1991; 198:1655–61.
18. Firth EC. Current concepts of infectious polyarthirtis in foals. Equine Vet J 1983; 15:5–9.

19. Vos NJ, Ducharme NG. Analysis of factors influencing prognosis in foals with septic arthritis. Irish Vet J 2008;61:102–6.
20. Bertone AL, Davis M, Cox HU. Arthrotomy versus arthroscopy and partial synovectomy for treatment of experimentally induced septic arthritis in horses. Am J Vet Res 1992;53:585–9.
21. Goodrich LR, Nixon AJ. Treatment options for osteomyelitis. Equine Vet Ed 2004; 16:267–80.
22. Smith LJ, Marr CM, Payne RJ. What is the likelihood that Thoroughbred foals treated for septic arthritis will race? Equine Vet J 2004;36:452–6.
23. Steel CM, Hunt AR, Adams PL, et al. Factors associated with prognosis for survival and athletic use in foals with septic arthritis. J Am Vet Med Assoc 1999; 215:973–7.

Prognostic Indicators for Survival and Athletic Outcome in Critically Ill Neonatal Foals

Pamela A. Wilkins, BS, DVM, MS, PhD

KEYWORDS

- L-Lactate • Sepsis • Prematurity • Neonatal encephalopathy • Critical care
- Intensive care

KEY POINTS

- Providing a prognosis for survival is generally more accurate than providing a prognosis for nonsurvival.
- Prognoses can be made for survival to hospital discharge, survival to a certain age, reaching certain sales expectations, or for performing as intended at a certain age among others.
- Many early studies were retrospective and focused on general populations of sick foals. More current prospective and retrospective studies are identifying differences in various prognostic indicators based on primary diagnostic categories, differences in management techniques, and changes in various indicators with time.
- No prognostic indicator will perform perfectly, particularly when dealing with a species where euthanasia decisions are commonly made for reasons other than impending death.

The management of critically ill foals is labor intensive, relatively expensive, and often stressful for the owner. Providing owners a well-informed prognosis for both survival and future usefulness of the foal early in the course of treatment is highly desirable. Today, there are many completed and ongoing projects aimed at improving the ability of equine practitioners to provide this information, but much work remains to be done. This article touches the surface of some of the indicators of outcomes that have been identified in order to provide the practitioner a sense of the utility of these indicators, particularly as they may relate to specific disease processes.

MATERNAL BODY WALL TEARS (PREPUBIC TENDON RUPTURES)

Early peer-reviewed reports of prepubic tendon and ventral body wall tears occurring in prepartum mares appeared in 1982 and 1986, respectively, although the conditions

The author has nothing to disclose.
Department of Veterinary Clinical Medicine, University of Illinois College of Veterinary Medicine, Urbana-Champaign, 1008 West Hazelwood Drive, IL 61801, USA
E-mail address: pawilkin@illinois.edu

were anecdotally known to veterinarians before that time.[1,2] The largest early reported case series described 4 mares with abdominal wall herniation and was published 30 years ago.[1] Three of the 4 cases in that case series were euthanized with no attempt to save the foal. The fourth case had parturition induced with delivery of a dead foal. The recommended treatment of abdominal wall herniation/prepubic tendon rupture was induction of parturition with attempts to save the foal depending on the owner's wishes and the supposed fetal readiness for birth.

Potential predisposing factors to body wall defects cited in the literature include hydrops allantois, hydrops amnion, trauma, twins, and fetal giants.[1,2] The earliest references suggested that mares be restricted to stall rest after induction, with abdominal support provided.[1] Repeat breeding was discouraged. Reported complications included laminitis, retained placenta, septic metritis, and shock.[2,3] Other primary literature pertaining to body wall defects focused on isolated cases.[4,5] Early reports suggested that mares be managed with supportive care, analgesia, restricted exercise, and abdominal support until they become suitable candidates for induction of parturition or elective cesarean section, carried out to prevent further abdominal wall trauma associated with abdominal muscle contraction during parturition yet allowing for potential delivery of a viable fetus.[1–4]

Treatment of mares with body wall defects has evolved over recent years at some facilities, and induction of parturition or elective cesarean section are generally avoided in these practices, when possible, because of potential risks to the fetus associated with inappropriate timing of induction of mares.[5,6] Conservative case management consists of stall rest/confinement, abdominal support, continuous monitoring of mare and fetus, and pain management, in addition to repeated ultrasonography and treatment of placentitis if indicated. All parturitions should be attended, and assistance rendered if necessary. Outcome for foals is improved with this conservative approach to management of body wall defects in pregnant mares compared with more interventional management approaches based on one recent study.[6] The study was a small, retrospective case series and, as such, has many limitations; however, it does serve to describe the conservative approach and allow reporting of outcomes using this approach.

Most importantly, the study showed that mares with body wall tear/prepubic tendon rupture could be successfully conservatively managed with a good prognosis for survival for the foal, making conservative management of mares with body wall defects the optimal therapeutic option, if possible, based on the condition of the dam. The outcome for mares did not seem to be significantly affected by type of management. Because few mares presented with hydrops allantois/amnion in the study, the investigators could not draw significant conclusions about the effects of hydrops allantois/amnion on mare survival, and although foal survival from mares with hydrops conditions has been reported, it is less in mares with hydrops conditions.[7] It is important to recognize that in some hydrops conditions, mares were euthanized shortly after presentation, or induced early in gestation, without attempt to save the fetus, introducing a bias based in clinician and owner perception of likelihood for survival that was not investigated. Despite the small number of cases reviewed, a clear improvement in outcome for foals was seen with conservative management of mares with body wall tear/prepubic tendon rupture, likely related to more appropriate readiness for birth. Not all cases are amenable to conservative management (ie, mares in extreme discomfort, or mares with rapidly enlarging body wall defects), and humane issues should always be of the primary concern for the attending clinician. However, mares with abdominal wall tear/prepubic tendon rupture can be successfully managed to term, and live, healthy foals can result from such pregnancies.

DYSTOCIA

Dystocia in the horse is a true emergency and threatens the lives of both the fetus and the dam. It has become increasing clear that time from onset of stage II labor until delivery directly impacts fetal survival. One report, from a large private equine referral practice in central Kentucky, evaluated outcome for mare and fetus based on time from onset of stage II to delivery and time from presentation at the referral hospital to delivery.[8] The mean difference in time from onset of dystocia to resolution between survivors and nonsurvivors for foals was less than 14 minutes. That study concluded that duration of dystocia has a profound effect on fetal survival and that resolution methods should be chosen to minimize this time duration.

A coordinated dystocia management protocol (CDMP) instituted in another referral hospital in 1997, used as a guideline for decision-making in an effort to decrease the time from presentation to dystocia resolution, was retrospectively examined in a 2006 report.[9] The purpose of that study was to evaluate the effects of instituting this CDMP on time to resolution and outcome for mare and foal. Institution of CDMP greatly decreased the time from presentation to resolution for mares presenting with dystocia on an emergency basis. However, the predicted time to resolution based on the protocol was shorter than the average time to resolution observed, and the protocol must be considered as a guideline for the decision-making process with room for improvement. The protocol was begun with the purpose of improving outcome for the fetus; unfortunately, this was not observed. Comorbidity, such as severe flexural deformity, and financial restriction played an important role in some cases. One explanation was uncovered in the continued prolonged time to presentation from onset of stage II labor before and after CDMP institution. The study demonstrated a large passage of time before hospital arrival, for most cases, that did not change after CDMP. Much of the delay before arrival was accounted for by travel distance and time spent before travel, possibly because of some owners/farm managers delaying the decision for referral or referring veterinarians/foaling personnel spending time attempting to correct the dystocia before referral. Other practical considerations, such as arranging transportation and familiarity, or lack thereof, of the route to the referral center, may also play a role and could not be evaluated in that study. Increased travel time and distance reflect a larger referral radius for dystocia in the later years and resulted in no change in overall duration of stage II labor despite less time spent in hospital resolving the dystocia. It is important to note that mare outcome was good to excellent in the study and that mare survival may dictate referral, even if fetal survival is unlikely.

The overall fetal survival-to-discharge rate from mares presenting with dystocia on an emergent basis was only 10% pre-CDMP and 13% post-CDMP, significantly less than the 23% overall survival reported from Kentucky.[8,9] In the Kentucky study, 70% of foals delivered alive survived to discharge. The percentage of foals delivered alive surviving to discharge in the second study was 30% and 43% pre-CDMP and post-CDMP, respectively, consistent with the prolonged duration before hospital arrival present in the more recent study. The time difference for total duration of stage II labor between foals delivered alive, and those not, was very large in the second study when compared with the Kentucky report.[8,9] The difference in live foal delivery percentage may be explained by the large difference in total stage II labor duration, as may be the difference in percentage of foals delivered alive that survived to discharge. It is very clear that duration of stage II labor directly impacts fetal survival, with an increased risk of nonsurvival to discharge of 16% for each 10-minute increase in stage II labor duration.

A recent retrospective report studied parturition, dystocia, and foal survival in 1047 births in a farm situation, perhaps a better indication of what to expect at a breeding farm when compared with a referral population.[10] Dystocia occurred in 10.1% of all births, and the incidence rate was higher in thoroughbred (TB) mares than in quarter horse mares. The most common cause of dystocia was abnormalities of fetal posture. A delay in foal delivery beyond 40 minutes of stage II of labor was associated with a significant increase in foal mortality, in agreement with the previous report.

Resolution of dystocia most commonly is accomplished by either assisted vaginal delivery or controlled vaginal delivery.[8,9] When cesarean section is required, there is an increase in dystocia duration, which directly impacts fetal survival. Early reports of cesarean section were associated with poor fetal survival, but also reported quite prolonged dystocia times.[11] Improved recognition of the need for cesarean section and rapid delivery of the fetus has importantly improved outcomes for the fetus, with an improved prognosis for delivery of a live foal if the duration of dystocia was less than 90 minutes and the dam less than 16 years of age.[12]

Overall, institution of dystocia protocols significantly decreases time from recognition to resolution for emergent dystocia cases. However, despite general knowledge that decreased dystocia duration translates to improved fetal survival, excessive or prolonged time before arrival at the hospital or site of definitive treatment will counteract any potential benefit the dystocia protocol may have on fetal survival, supporting the development of dystocia protocols at breeding farms. Dystocia remains an emergency condition of the mare and prompt relief at the farm—or referral, either immediately or once dystocia is recognized to be challenging—should result in improved fetal survival. Time is life for the fetus.

L-LACTATE

Increased blood or plasma L-lactate concentration ([LAC]) is commonly associated with disease severity and mortality and is a neonatal equine emergency.[13–19] Increased disease severity and mortality of patients with hyperlactemia remain a persistent feature of many diseases of foals regardless of whether [LAC] was evaluated as a single, one-time measurement or sequentially over a period of time. Although initial concentrations of LAC at birth are expected because of fetal metabolism, these values should decrease rapidly and be within the adult normal range between 3 and 5 days following birth.[20–22] The role of [LAC] as a biomarker and the association with clinical disease is complex, and these questions remain: why do patients with increased [LAC] die more frequently than patients without increased [LAC], and, are there problems of neonatal foals where increased [LAC] is more specifically associated with nonsurvival?

The objective of one recent study was to investigate the association [LAC]$_{ADMIT}$ with presenting complaint, periparturient events, outcome, and clinical diagnosis in a prospective multicenter approach and also investigate the association of hyperlactemia with some historical periparturient events, presenting complaints, and clinical diagnoses.[13] This study of 643 foals presented an opportunity to evaluate overall survival and outcome data, in addition to evaluating categorical survival by periparturient history, presenting complaint and clinical diagnostic category, in critically ill foals presenting for veterinary care at referral hospitals without regard to [LAC]$_{ADMIT}$. Overall survival rate was 79%. Nonsurvivors included foals euthanized for poor prognosis determined by the clinician (N = 81) or financial reasons (N = 6). Forty-eight foals died. Mean age at admission was 53 ± 16 hours (range 0–840 hours) and was not significantly different between survivors and nonsurvivors. Gestational age varied significantly between survivors and nonsurvivors (339 ± 15 days vs 331 ± 16 days). Foals born from known dystocia, even if not the major clinical diagnosis for the foal, had significantly larger [LAC]$_{ADMIT}$ than foals without known dystocia (6.9 ± 4.4 mmol/L vs 4.9 ± 4.4 mmol/L). The same was true for foals born following recognized premature placental separation compared with those without (7.8 ± 5.8 mmol/L vs 4.9 ± 4.1 mmol/L).

The most common presenting complaint was diarrhea (91% survival) followed by "dummy" foal (77% survival), recumbency (80% survival), cesarean section/dystocia/high-risk pregnancy (78% survival), colic (86% survival), lethargy (89% survival), not nursing (89% survival), premature (54% survival), orthopedic problems (77% survival), suspected sepsis (60% survival), colostral-related problems (94% survival), respiratory problems (93% survival), umbilical-related problems (93% survival), trauma (73% survival), FPT/requiring blood transfusion (91% survival), rejected by mare (100% survival), uroperitoneum (100% survival), meconium impaction (100% survival), neurologic/seizures (100% survival), and dysphagia (100% survival).

After admission and diagnostic testing, foals were placed in 1 of 18 final clinical diagnosis groups based on which most represented the primary problem determined by the attending clinician: perinatal asphyxia syndrome (survival 88%), unspecified diarrhea (survival 93%), sepsis (survival 59%), and prematurity/dysmaturity (survival 53%) were the most frequent diagnoses, followed by other (survival 69%), meconium impaction (survival 100%), failure of passive transfer (FPT) (survival 100%), unspecified colic (survival 75%), unspecified trauma (survival 72%), orthopedic problems (survival 68%), immunologic problems/neonatal isoerythrolysis other than FPT (survival 94%), respiratory (survival 42%), uroperitoneum (survival 73%), high-risk pregnancy/dystocia (survival 100%), dysphagia (survival 78%), unspecified congenital deformity (survival 17%), muscle disease (survival 100%), and umbilical disease not related to uroperitoneum (survival 100%).

Admission blood culture results were available for 72.5% of foals, with 74.2% reported as negative and 25.8% reported as positive. Fifty-three (44.2%) isolates were gram-positive, whereas 73 (60.8%) were gram-negative isolates. Positive blood culture was significantly associated with negative outcome; however, [LAC]$_{ADMIT}$ was not significantly different in blood culture–positive versus –negative foals when considered over the entire study population (5.3 ± 4.6 mmol/L vs 5.0 ± 3.9 mmol/L).

Median [LAC]$_{ADMIT}$ was significantly increased in nonsurvivors compared with survivors in those foals where it was measured (n = 586/643; 91.1%). Median and mean [LAC]$_{ADMIT}$ were both different and associated with different risk of nonsurvival (odds ratio) between final diagnosis groups. Six clinicians' major diagnoses had increased odds of nonsurvival for each 1 mmol/L increase in [LAC]$_{ADMIT}$: sepsis; unspecified enterocolitis; unspecified colic; unspecified trauma; immune related (not FPT), and respiratory-only.

The most important finding of the study was the overall large survival rate of foals presenting to neonatal intensive care units (NICUs) throughout the world, in addition to the uniformity of that survival rate across multiple centers providing such care. This overall large survival rate is certainly a positive finding and should encourage those engaged in the practice of neonatal intensive care, both practitioners and owners, to pursue treatment when financially acceptable. Regarding the direct intent of the study, it confirmed the findings of several smaller studies that [LAC]$_{ADMIT}$ is associated with outcome. Uniquely, multicenter prospective study strongly suggested that the utility of [LAC]$_{ADMIT}$ as a prognostic indicator is greater in certain clinical diagnostic categories than in others in the equine neonate.

The longstanding concept that LAC is a biomarker that may accurately predict morbidity and mortality when [LAC] is evaluated as a single admission measurement holds true for this prospective multicenter study, as [LAC]$_{ADMIT}$ was significantly higher in nonsurvivors on initial admission. This concept is in agreement with previous studies but carries greater weight by being both prospective and multicenter in design. Of interest is the observation that large [LAC] at admission does not necessarily translate to poorer outcome, but rather is potentially a better performing biomarker within specific major diagnosis categories. This observation may explain the finding that admission [LAC] generally allows only ~80% of foals to be correctly classified as survivors or nonsurvivors based on [LAC]$_{ADMIT}$ alone. Although useful, [LAC]$_{ADMIT}$ should not be used as a single determinant of prognosis, but rather as part of the overall picture—including major clinical diagnosis—when advising clients and trying to establish an accurate prognosis. There are clear differences in the interpretation of [LAC]$_{ADMIT}$ based on the clinician determination of major clinically important diagnoses that should be considered when using [LAC]$_{ADMIT}$ as a prognostic indicator. There is interest in evaluating a new LAC measure, the area under the [LAC] versus time curve for the first 24 hours following admission, with normal values for foals reported and a preliminary prospective multicenter study reporting differences between surviving and nonsurviving foals.[22,23]

GLUCOSE

Hypoglycemia in critically ill foals at admission has been correlated with nonsurvival to hospital discharge in septic foals, and with survival to 96 hours—but not to hospital discharge—in foals presenting to NICUs.[24] There is general clinical acceptance that hyperglycemia is also common in critically ill foals, but its prevalence and association with outcome have not been well documented. A fairly recent multicenter retrospective study of blood glucose concentrations in critically ill foals investigated blood glucose concentrations in 515 critically ill neonatal horses at admission and for the first 60 hours of hospitalization, to determine if there was a measurable association of blood glucose concentrations with survival, sepsis, and the systemic inflammatory response syndrome (SIRS) critically ill neonatal foals.[24] Hypoglycemia (glucose ≤75 mg/dL) at admission was associated with poorer survival to hospital discharge, and each 18 mg/dL increase in blood glucose increased the odds of survival to hospital discharge more than 3-fold. Hypoglycemia at admission was associated with sepsis, SIRS, and positive blood culture. Low to moderate hyperglycemia (blood glucose >131 mg/dL but <180 mg/dL) did not have similar associations. Extreme hyperglycemia (blood glucose >180 mg/dL) was associated with a poorer prognosis to hospital discharge as was extreme hypoglycemia (blood glucose <50 mg/dL) at admission when compared with those with blood glucose concentrations greater than 50.4 mg/dL. Extreme hypoglycemia was also associated with sepsis and positive blood culture but not with SIRS. Blood glucose concentrations at 48 hours or any time point after 48 hours of hospitalization showed no association with survival to hospital discharge. This study suggests that both hypoglycemia and extreme hyperglycemia at admission may be useful prognostic indicators. The reader is cautioned that glucose derangements likely serve primarily as indicators of disease severity and, similar to [LAC]$_{ADMIT}$, are not necessarily the direct cause of nonsurvival. Aberrant glucose values need to be corrected, but, more importantly, the underlying and root causes need to be treated and resolved.

MUSCULOSKELETAL

A significant proportion of foals will be born with either flexural or angular limb deformities. There are very few reports regarding outcome and racing performance in affected foals, although a few studies exist reporting on therapies developed in the 1980s and 1990s. One such study suggested that desmotomy of the accessory liga- ment of the deep digital flexor muscle (inferior check desmotomy) performed at an early age allowed standardbred (SB) foals with flexural deformities to reach the racetrack.[25] Twenty-three SBs were studied over 10 years. Six of 11 foals treated sur- gically either raced 6 times and obtained a race record or were training sound at the study was published. All 12 horses that did not have surgical intervention had no record of racing. No foals treated surgically after 8 months of age had a good outcome. This surgery is no longer commonly performed on foals with congenital flex- ural deformities because medical treatment with oxytetracycline and physical ther- apy—or devices designed specifically for those purposes—are more commonly used with anecdotal clinical success.[26–29]

Many foals are affected by angular limb deformities, and surgical correction is still indicated in some severe cases not responding to medical management.[30–34] However, many foals have undergone procedures such as hemicircumferential perios- teal transection and elevation ("stripping") that were not strictly necessary, because most of mild or even moderate cases resolve with maturity and increased lateral medial stability of the carpus or other affected joints.[31,34] There is one early report sug- gesting that although there are differences related to surgery and sex between affected/treated foals and controls related to reaching the track, these differences did not translate into fewer starts, wins, or earnings over their careers once at the track.[32]

Septic arthritis is a serious problem in the foal and carries a poor prognosis for both short-term survival, primarily associated with concurrent serious disease or multiple sites of infection, and surviving as an athletic horse. A retrospective study of 93 foals with septic arthritis reviewed medical records and race records for TB and SB foals in order to evaluate athletic outcome for these breeds.[35] Seventy-eight percent survived to hospital discharge, with ~33% of the study foals racing. The prognosis for survival of foals with septic arthritis was favorable; however, the prognosis for racing (and good performance while racing) was not. Systemic disease other than the musculoskeletal system, joint infection with *Salmonella* spp, multiple affected joints, and synovial fluid neutrophil percentage greater than or equal to 95% at admission seemed to be of prognostic value, although not quantitated.

In a 2004 report, medical records of 69 foals treated for septic arthritis were reviewed.[36] The lifetime racing records for the affected foals and at least one sibling was reviewed, and the investigators reported that foals with septic arthritis were at least 3 times less likely to start on a racecourse compared with controls. Again, systemic disease in additional to the musculoskeletal system was associated with an approximate 8-fold decreased likelihood of surviving. However, those surviving hospitalization were as likely as their siblings to start in at least one race. Foals dis- charged following treatment of septic arthritis were significantly older when starting the first time compared with siblings. These investigators concluded that development of septic arthritis in a TB foal significantly reduced the likelihood of starting on a racecourse.

With several retrospective studies evaluating the factors associated with prognosis in foals with septic arthritis, it seems that the presence of concurrent osteomyelitis negatively influences prognosis, with epiphyseal lesions and multiple joint involve- ment predicting poor survival to discharge and athletic outcome. The prognostic value of variables found in septic bony lesions (osteomyelitis) has received less atten- tion until recently, when a retrospective study of 108 foals with osteomyelitis reported on the clinical characteristics, short-term survival, and future athletic performance of that population.[37] Approximately 20% of foals with osteomyelitis had radiographically apparent lesions in multiple locations, whereas ~70% had concurrent septic arthritis. As seen with more modern studies evaluating bacterial isolates in sepsis, isolated bacteria were fairly evenly split between gram-negative and gram-positive isolates, neither more associated with decreased likelihood of racing. As observed in multiple studies of sick neonatal foals, younger age, concurrent diseases, and multiple affected joints were associated with decreased survival hospital discharge. Eighty-one percent of affected foals were discharged (80.6%), with 91% of survivors achieving racing age and 60% of those starting. The most frequently affected bones were the femur (~25%), tibia (~22%), and distal phalanx (~20%). Foals with P-type (ospteomyelitis of the physis) lesions were 4.7 times more likely to race, whereas those with both P- and E-type (osteomyelitis of the epiphysis) lesions were significantly less likely to race, and those with P/E-type lesions of the tibia were even less likely to race. Overall, 48% of the foals treated for osteomyelitis (survivors and nonsurvivors included) raced. Similar to others, the investigators reported that the prognosis for survival of foals with septic osteomyelitis or osteitis is good, unless complicated by other disease states or multiple bone/joint disease. This study was the first to report that foals surviving multiple infected bone sites—without multiple joint involvement—had a good prognosis for racing, although certainly less than unaffected foals. In addition, one racing performance was not different from the overall TB population, according to mean earnings reported by the Australian Stud Book.

The short-term survival rate for one neonatal intensive care unit (NICU) between 1990 and 1995 was 80.8% for 287 racing breed foals compared with a control cohort of siblings in one report.[38] The attrition rate of NICU survivors before registration was higher, and the number of registered NICU survivors with more than one race start was lower than the control population. Fifty-nine percent of TB and 44% of the SB foals discharged from the NICU had more than one race start. There were no significant differences in the earnings, number of starts, earnings/start, and places/start over the first 2-year period of racing between the NICU survivors with more than one race start and their controls, suggesting that, overall, once survivors make it to the track they do well. However, NICU survivors with perinatal asphyxia syndrome ("dummy foals"), generalized sepsis, and localized infectious disease had significantly lower earnings in their first year of racing than their controls. Premature/immature NICU survivors had significantly fewer places and earnings per start over the 2-year period than their controls. These findings support the concept that the prognosis for athletic (racing) outcome varies by primary disease condition, as does the prognosis for survival. Currently, there are no similar studies for other endeavors of athletic horses, difficult to perform because a lack of objective outcome data measures.

Many racing breed foals are intended to be sold at public auction. The impact of disease conditions necessitating hospital treatment as a foal on future sales performance is unknown. In one recent study, foals aged less than 125 days surviving treatment at a hospital and presented for sale at public auction were evaluated.[39] Sales outcomes of the NICU foals were compared with those of 6 controls for each subject: 3 horses immediately prior and 3 horses immediately following the subject at the same sale. Sixty-three previously hospitalized foals went to public auction: 19 at foal sales, 39 at yearling sales, and 5 at 2-year-old sales. Forty-five (71%) sold, not different from controls. No difference was found in mean sales price. The investigators concluded that, overall, hospitalization and treatment of TB foals had no impact on sales outcome for survivors presenting to public auction. They did not report on the percentage of NICU foals intended for sale that went to sale.

RESPIRATORY

There are several studies available that looked at prognostic indicators for neonatal foals with a variety of forms of respiratory disease.[40–45] Two studies from 2003 took advantage of a group of 163 neonatal foals with thoracic radiographs taken within 48 hours of admission to a referral hospital.[40,41] The objectives of the first was to identify risk factors for the development of thoracic radiographic changes and to identify prognostic indicators for survival in foals with radiographic evidence of pulmonary disease. Failure of transfer of passive immunity was the only risk factor for radiographic evidence of respiratory disease identified by multivariate analysis. Hypoxemic patients (P_aO_2 ≤60 mm Hg) were 4.9 times more likely to have radiographic changes. Foals with a serum creatinine concentration greater than 1.7 mg/dL, dyspnea, and a history of dystocia at presentation were significantly more likely to die. An anion gap (poor man's lactate) greater than or equal to 20 mEq/dL was strongly associated with nonsurvival and seemed to have the greatest clinical importance. Most physical examination variables, surprising at the time, were unrelated to outcome. The second related study evaluated 207 thoracic radiographs from 128 foals to investigate potential associations between pulmonary radiographic pattern, distribution, and severity of pulmonary changes and short-term survival of neonatal foals. Not surprisingly, dyspneic foals had more extensive pulmonary infiltrates within the cranioventral lung, more advanced respiratory disease, and lower survival rates. Tachypnea most consistently related to diffuse (caudodorsal, caudoventral, and cranioventral) pulmonary changes. A fibrinogen concentration greater than 400 mg/dL was associated with increased cranioventral radiographic abnormalities, whereas neutropenia, milk reflux from the nares, upper airway abnormality, abnormal respiratory sounds, failure of transfer of passive immunity (immunoglobulin G concentration <400 mg/dL), immaturity, or fever were not related to radiographic pattern, distribution, or severity of radiographic changes. Sixty-five percent of foals with radiographic pulmonary disease were discharged alive. Increased caudodorsal radiographic score was significantly associated with nonsurvival, with potential as a prognostic indicator because of increased association with equine neonatal acute lung injury and equine neonatal acute respiratory distress syndrome.

Rhodococcus equi bronchopneumonia and related problems affect a large proportion of foals worldwide. Treatment and management changes have been investigated and are commonly used on farms where the disease is endemic. In racing breeds, there is always a concern that a severe pulmonary infection, such as *R equi*, could be fatal or career ending. Two studies from the mid-1990s evaluated the impact of *R equi* on persistent radiographic abnormalities following survival and then racing performance.[42,43] The purpose of the studies were to determine whether physical examination, laboratory, or radiographic abnormalities in foals with *R equi* infection were associated with survival, ability to race at least once after recovery, or, for foals that survived and went on to race, subsequent racing performance. In these multicenter retrospective studies, 49 TB and 66 SBs diagnosed with *R equi* infection were evaluated. Eighty-three (72%) foals survived. Foals that did not survive were more likely to have extreme tachycardia (heart rate >100 beats/min) and respiratory distress and to have severe radiographic abnormalities at the time of initial examination. There were no clinicopathologic abnormalities associated with survival. Forty-five of the 83 surviving foals (54%) eventually raced at least once, but none of the factors examined was associated with whether foals raced. Racing performance of foals that raced as adults was not different from that of the general US racing population. *R equi* infection in foals seems to be associated with a decreased likelihood of racing; however, surviving foals that do race perform comparably to the general US racing population.

A syndrome resembling acute lung injury (ALI)/acute respiratory distress syndrome (ARDS) was described in 23 foals, between 1 and 7 months old, in the early 1990s.[44] Characteristic features included sudden onset of severe respiratory distress and tachypnea, cyanosis unresponsive to nasal oxygen, pyrexia, hypoxemia, hypercapneic respiratory acidosis, poor response to treatment, and histopathologic lesions of bronchiolitis and bronchointerstitial pneumonia. Very few foals survived, and those that did were treated with corticosteroids in addition to broad-spectrum antimicrobials and other supportive therapies. It was not until 2008 that a veterinary definition for these conditions was established.[45] Because so few reports exist in the veterinary medical literature describing clinical and pathologic findings resembling conditions described of ALI and ARDS, a study was undertaken early the 2000s to document history, clinical, laboratory, and diagnostic findings, treatment, and outcome of foals age 1 to 12 months diagnosed with ALI/ARDS at a referral hospital.[46] Radiographic, cytologic, microbiological, serologic, and postmortem findings were reviewed to identify foals with acute onset of respiratory distress, a partial pressure of arterial oxygen (P_aO_2) to fraction of oxygen in inspired gases (Fio_2) ratio of less than or equal to 300 mm Hg, pulmonary infiltrates on thoracic radiographs, and postmortem findings consistent with ALI/ARDS. Fifteen foals age 1.5 to 8 months were included in the study. All foals developed acute respiratory distress less than 48 hours before presentation. Tachycardia and tachypnea were consistently present, with fever recorded in 8 cases. Eight cases met the criteria for ALI (P_aO_2 to Fio_2 ratio $\leq$300 mm Hg) and 7 for ARDS (P_aO_2 to Fio_2 ratio $\leq$200 mm Hg). Radiographic findings demonstrated diffuse bronchointerstitial pattern with focal to coalescing alveolar radiopacities. An infectious cause was identified in 10 foals. All foals were treated with intranasal oxygen and antimicrobial drugs; 13 received corticosteroids. Nine foals survived; 4 died due to respiratory failure, and 2 were subjected to euthanasia in a moribund state. Follow-up was available for 7 surviving foals; all performed as well as age mates or siblings, and one raced successfully. The investigators concluded that a condition similar to ALI/ARDS in humans exists in foals age 1 to 12 months and may be identical to previously described acute bronchointerstitial pneumonia in young horses. Although prognosis may appear poor for survival, treatment with systemic corticosteroids, intranasal oxygen, and antimicrobials appears beneficial in foals with clinical signs compatible with ALI/ARDS. Surviving foals, although only small numbers have been documented, appear to do well and perform as expected later in life.

THE FUTURE
Coagulation Testing

Traditional and viscoelastic coagulation testing had become more commonly performed at large referral hospitals, but the utility of these tests is still being evaluated. One study prospectively evaluated changes in viscoelastic variables looking for any associations with abnormalities observed in the standard coagulation profile and patient outcome in foals with suspected sepsis.[47] The study enrolled 30 critically ill foals less than 72-hours-old admitted sequentially that met criteria for SIRS associated with infection. Foals with decreasing clot rate over the sample period were more likely to be euthanized or die. Identification of coagulopathy on admission, or persistence of hemostatic dysfunction 48 hours later, was associated with death. The investigators suggested that viscoelastic coagulation testing could be used in an

NICU setting to further characterize coagulopathy and identify foals at higher risk for poor outcome.

Another prospective study of standard coagulation parameters in 63 foals classified as septic shock, septic, and other found at least 1 abnormal value in 18 of 28 (64%) samples from the septic shock group, 66 of 85 (78%) from the septic group, and 30 of 59 (51%) from the other group.[48,49] Coagulopathy (3 or more abnormal values) was present in 25% of samples in the septic shock group, 16% of samples in the septic group, and 5% of samples in the other group. Foals in septic shock were 12.7 times more likely to have clinical evidence of bleeding than those in the other group (95% confidence interval 2.3–70, P = .004). The investigators concluded that coagulopathy commonly occurs in critically ill neonatal foals, especially those with sepsis and septic shock, but did not indicate an increased risk of nonsurvival associated with any specific abnormality.

SUMMARY

There is one article that demonstrates a key point: the good clinician just knows. The group created a mathematical model to assist in the early prediction of probability of survival in hospitalized foals less than 7 days of age.[50] It was a prospective multicenter design that evaluated data from 1073 foals. Data, 34 variables, were collected from the medical records of 910 hospitalized foals to develop the model, and the variables associated being discharged alive were entered into a multivariate logistic regression model. The model was then validated prospectively on data from an additional 163 foals. Clinicians responsible for the cases were asked shortly after admission if they thought the foal would survive or not. Factors in the final model included age, ability to stand, presence of suckle reflex, white blood cell count, serum creatinine concentration, and anion gap (remember, this is poor man's [LAC]). Sensitivity and specificity of the model to predict survival to discharge were 92% and 74%, respectively, in the retrospective population, and 90% and 46%, respectively, in the prospective population. Accuracy of an equine clinician's initial prediction of the foal being discharged alive was 83%, and accuracy of the model's prediction was 81%. Combining the clinician's prediction of probability of live discharge with that of the model significantly increased (median increase, 12%) the accuracy of the prediction for foals that were discharged and nonsignificantly decreased (median decrease, 9%) the accuracy of the predication for nonsurvivors.

Combining the clinician's initial predication of the probability of a foal being discharged alive with that of the model seemed to provide a more precise early estimate of the probability of live discharge for hospitalized foals than the model alone! However, we are better at predicting survival than nonsurvival; this is probably related to intangible and immeasurable factors: owner's tolerance, financial consideration, perception, and history with previous sick foals or those who had sick foals. Because there is the option of euthanasia for many reasons, including clinician's or owner's perception of poor prognosis and financial/value driven reasons, the data will always be a bit "muddy."

REFERENCES

1. Jackson PG. Rupture of the prepubic tendon in a shire mare. Vet Rec 1982; 111(2):38.
2. Hanson RR, Todhunter RJ. Herniation of the abdominal wall in pregnant mares. J Am Vet Med Assoc 1986;189(7):790–3.

3. Perkins NR, Frazer GS. Reproductive emergencies in the mare. Vet Clin North Am Equine Pract 1994;10(3):643–70.
4. Mirza MH, Paccamonti D, Martin GS, et al. Theriogenology question of the month. Rupture of the prepubic tendon with additional tearing of the abdominal tunic. J Am Vet Med Assoc 1997;211(10):1237–8.
5. Seyrek-Intas K, Kumru IH, Seyrek-Intas D. Rupture of the prepubic tendon in a congenitally lordotic mare. Tierarztl Prax Ausg G Grosstiere Nutztiere 2011; 39(1):46–8.
6. Ross J, Palmer JE, Wilkins PA. Body wall tears during late pregnancy in mares: 13 cases (1995-2006). J Am Vet Med Assoc 2008;232(2):257–61.
7. Christensen BW, Troedsson MH, Murchie TA, et al. Management of hydrops amnion in a mare resulting in birth of a live foal. J Am Vet Med Assoc 2006; 228(8):1228–33.
8. Byron CR, Embertson RM, Bernard WV, et al. Dystocia in a referral hospital setting: approach and results. Equine Vet J 2003;35(1):82–5.
9. Norton JL, Dallap BL, Johnston JK, et al. Retrospective study of dystocia in mares at a referral hospital. Equine Vet J 2007;39(1):37–41.
10. McCue PM, Ferris RA. Parturition, dystocia and foal survival: a retrospective study of 1047 births. Equine Vet J Suppl 2012;(41):22–5 [Erratum in Equine Vet J Suppl 2013;45(2):259].
11. Freeman DE, Hungerford LL, Schaeffer D, et al. Caesarean section and other methods for assisted delivery: comparison of effects on mare mortality and complications. Equine Vet J 1999;31(3):203–7.
12. Abernathy-Young KK, LeBlanc MM, Embertson RM, et al. Survival rates of mares and foals and postoperative complications and fertility of mares after cesarean section: 95 cases (1986-2000). J Am Vet Med Assoc 2012;241(7):927–34.
13. Borchers A, Wilkins PA, Marsh PM, et al. Association of admission L-lactate concentration in hospitalised equine neonates with presenting complaint, peripartur-ient events, clinical diagnosis and outcome: a prospective multicentre study. Equine Vet J 2012;(Suppl 41):57–63.
14. Borchers A, Wilkins PA, Marsh PM, et al. Sequential L-lactate concentration in hospitalized equine neonates: a prospective multicenter study. Equine Vet J 2013;(45):2–7.
15. Castagnetti C, Pirrone A, Mariella J, et al. Venous blood lactate evaluation in equine neonatal intensive care. Theriogenology 2010;73:343–57.
16. Corley KTT, Donaldson LL, Furr MO. Arterial lactate concentration, hospital survival, sepsis, and SIRS in critically ill neonatal foals. Equine Vet J 2005;37:53–9.
17. Henderson ISF, Franklin RP, Wilkins PA, et al. Association of hyperlactemia with age, diagnosis, and survival in equine neonates. J Vet Emerg Crit Care 2008; 18:496–502.
18. Wotman K, Wilkins PA, Palmer JE, et al. Association of blood lactate concentration and outcome in foals. J Vet Intern Med 2009;23:598–605.
19. Magdesian KG. Blood lactate levels in neonatal foals: normal values and temporal effects in the post-partum period [abstract]. J Vet Emerg Crit Care 2003;13(2):174.
20. Père MC. Materno-fetal exchanges and utilization of nutrients by the fetus: comparison between species. Reprod Nutr Dev 2003;43(1):1–15.
21. Pirrone A, Mariella J, Gentilini F, et al. Amniotic fluid and blood lactate concentrations in mares and foals in the early postpartum period. Theriogenology 2012; 78(6):1182–9.
22. Sheahan B, Wilkins PA, Lascola KM, et al. L-Lactate area (LACArea) in neonatal foals from birth to 14 days of age. J Vet Emerg Crit Care, in press.

23. Wilkins PA, Sheahan BJ, Vander Werf KA, et al. Preliminary investigation of the area under the L-lactate concentration-time curve (LACArea) in critically ill equine neonate. J Vet Intern Med 2015;29(2):659–62.
24. Hollis AR, Furr MO, Magdesian KG, et al. Blood glucose concentrations in critically ill neonatal foals. J Vet Intern Med 2008;22(5):1223–7.
25. Stick JA, Nickels FA, Williams MA. Long-term effects of desmotomy of the accessory ligament of the deep digital flexor muscle in standardbreds: 23 cases (1979-1989). J Am Vet Med Assoc 1992;200(8):1131–2.
26. Madison JB, Garber JL, Rice B, et al. Effect of oxytetracycline on metacarpophalangeal and distal interphalangeal joint angles in newborn foals. J Am Vet Med Assoc 1994;204(2):246–9.
27. Kasper CA, Clayton HM, Wright AK, et al. Effects of high doses of oxytetracycline on metacarpophalangeal joint kinematics in neonatal foals. J Am Vet Med Assoc 1995;207(1):71–3.
28. Arnoczky SP, Lavagnino M, Gardner KL, et al. In vitro effects of oxytetracycline on matrix metalloproteinase-1 mRNA expression and on collagen gel contraction by cultured myofibroblasts obtained from the accessory ligament of foals. Am J Vet Res 2004;65(4):491–6.
29. Wintz LR, Lavagnino M, Gardner KL, et al. Age-dependent effects of systemic administration of oxytetracycline on the viscoelastic properties of rat tail tendons as a mechanistic basis for pharmacological treatment of flexural limb deformities in foals. Am J Vet Res 2012;73(12):1951–6.
30. O'Donohue DD, Smith FH, Strickland KL. The incidence of abnormal limb development in the Irish thoroughbred from birth to 18 months. Equine Vet J 1992; 24(4):305–9.
31. Robert C, Valette JP, Denoix JM. Longitudinal development of equine forelimb conformation from birth to weaning in three different horse breeds. Vet J 2013; 198(Suppl 1):e75–80.
32. Mitten LA, Bramlage LR, Embertson RM. Racing performance after hemicircumferential periosteal transection for angular limb deformities in thoroughbreds: 199 cases (1987-1989). J Am Vet Med Assoc 1995;207(6):746–50.
33. Dutton DM, Watkins JP, Honnas CM, et al. Treatment response and athletic outcome of foals with tarsal valgus deformities: 39 cases (1988-1997). J Am Vet Med Assoc 1999;215(10):1481–4.
34. Read EK, Read MR, Townsend HG, et al. Effect of hemi-circumferential periosteal transection and elevation in foals with experimentally induced angular limb deformities. J Am Vet Med Assoc 2002;221(4):536–40.
35. Steel CM, Hunt AR, Adams PL, et al. Factors associated with prognosis for survival and athletic use in foals with septic arthritis: 93 cases (1987-1994). J Am Vet Med Assoc 1999;215(7):973–7.
36. Smith LJ, Marr CM, Payne RJ, et al. What is the likelihood that thoroughbred foals treated for septic arthritis will race? Equine Vet J 2004;36(5):452–6.
37. Neil KM, Axon JE, Begg AP, et al. Retrospective study of 108 foals with septic osteomyelitis. Aust Vet J 2010;88(1–2):4–12.
38. Axon J, Palmer J, Wilkins P. Short- and long-term athletic outcome of neonatal intensive care unit survivors. Proc Am Assoc Equine Pract 1999;46:224–5.
39. Corley KT, Corley MM. Hospital treatment as a foal does not adversely affect future sales performance in thoroughbred horses. Equine Vet J Suppl 2012;41:87–90.
40. Bedenice D, Heuwieser W, Solano M, et al. Risk factors and prognostic variables for survival of foals with radiographic evidence of pulmonary disease. J Vet Intern Med 2003;17(6):868–75.

41. Bedenice D, Heuwieser W, Brawer R, et al. Clinical and prognostic significance of radiographic pattern, distribution, and severity of thoracic radiographic changes in neonatal foals. J Vet Intern Med 2003;17(6):876–86.
42. Ainsworth DM, Beck KA, Boatwright CE, et al. Lack of residual lung damage in horses in which Rhodococcus equi-induced pneumonia had been diagnosed. Am J Vet Res 1993;54(12):2115–20.
43. Ainsworth DM, Eicker SW, Yeagar AE, et al. Associations between physical examination, laboratory, and radiographic findings and outcome and subsequent racing performance of foals with Rhodococcus equi infection: 115 cases (1984-1992). J Am Vet Med Assoc 1998;213(4):510–5.
44. Lakritz J, Wilson WD, Berry CR, et al. Bronchointerstitial pneumonia and respiratory distress in young horses: clinical, clinicopathologic, radiographic, and pathological findings in 23 cases (1984-1989). J Vet Intern Med 1993;7(5):277–88.
45. Wilkins PA, Otto CM, Dunkel B, et al. Acute lung injury (ALI) and acute respiratory distress syndromes (ARDS) in veterinary medicine: consensus definitions. J Vet Emerg Crit Care 2007;17(4):333–9.
46. Dunkel B, Dolente B, Boston RC. Acute lung injury/acute respiratory distress syndrome in 15 foals. Equine Vet J 2005;37(5):435–40.
47. Dallap Schaer BL, Epstein K. Coagulopathy of the critically ill equine patient. J Vet Emerg Crit Care 2009;19(1):53–65.
48. Bentz AI, Palmer JE, Dallap BL, et al. Prospective evaluation of coagulation in critically ill neonatal foals. J Vet Intern Med 2009;23(1):161–7.
49. Dallap Schaer BL, Bentz AI, Boston RC, et al. Comparison of viscoelastic coagulation analysis and standard coagulation profiles in critically ill neonatal foals to outcome. J Vet Emerg Crit Care 2009;19(1):88–95.
50. Rohrbach BW, Buchanan BR, Drake JM, et al. Use of a multivariable model to estimate the probability of discharge in hospitalized foals that are 7 days of age or less. J Am Vet Med Assoc 2006;228(11):1748–56.

Index

Note: Page numbers of article titles are in **boldface** type.

Vet Clin Equine 31 (2015) 629–638
http://dx.doi.org/10.1016/S0749-0739(15)00074-7
0749-0739/15/$ – see front matter © 2015 Elsevier Inc. All rights reserved.

vetequine.theclinics.com

Moving?

Make sure your subscription moves with you!

To notify us of your new address, find your **Clinics Account Number** (located on your mailing label above your name), and contact customer service at:

Email: journalscustomerservice-usa@elsevier.com

800-654-2452 (subscribers in the U.S. & Canada)
314-447-8871 (subscribers outside of the U.S. & Canada)

Fax number: 314-447-8029

**Elsevier Health Sciences Division
Subscription Customer Service
3251 Riverport Lane
Maryland Heights, MO 63043**

*To ensure uninterrupted delivery of your subscription, please notify us at least 4 weeks in advance of move.

Printed and bound by CPI Group (UK) Ltd, Croydon, CR0 4YY

03/10/2024

01040494-0017